Lisa Morse
MS, RDN, CNSC

Arizona State University

INTERPROFESSIONAL APPROACH to ASSESSMENT *from a* NUTRITIONAL PERSPECTIVE

Kendall Hunt
publishing company

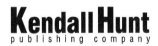

www.kendallhunt.com
Send all inquiries to:
4050 Westmark Drive
Dubuque, IA 52004-1840

Contents

Introduction

The clinical assessment of a patient or client is based on both science and art. Practitioners rely on published standards to evaluate a patient and determine the best course of therapeutic action. Both subjective data from the patient's perspective and objective data are utilized to determine the best overall intervention for the particular patient circumstances. Over time, as research changes so do evaluation standards and therapeutic recommendations. Each practitioner will use published standards but may interpret them slightly different, so some subjective information from the practitioner's perspective may be introduced as well. This is where the art of assessment comes into play.

Science determines current standards of care. Critical thinking skills will determine how to use the actual standards and this is the art of assessment. A practitioner does not always have to, or want to implement an intervention any time a piece of data is outside the normal limits of a standard. The practitioner must use critical thinking skills to determine how far outside the published standard will be considered acceptable for a particular patient or in a particular set of circumstances. These acceptable conditions or circumstances are fluid and changing. Critical thinking skills allow evaluation of ever-changing circumstances to determine the best possible therapy for the best possible patient outcome at any given time. Rarely is there only one correct answer in the evaluation of these many complex pieces of data. Relying on the advice from experts in specific areas (e.g., endocrinology, dietetics, and pharmacy) may be necessary to provide the best possible care for a patient or client. Different practitioners or even different individuals working in the same area of expertise may view these sets of data differently and come up with slightly different recommendations for the same patient. Interprofessional discussion and evaluation from these different perspectives will allow expansion of knowledge and ongoing evaluation of standards of care.

It is important to note that each set of unique circumstances for each patient or client creates a unique set of data to evaluate. Not all data are pertinent and not all data must be addressed. Intervention may not need to be implemented on every piece of data that is outside the normal limits. The art of critical thinking will help the practitioner determine what needs to be addressed now, what can wait until later, and what is not pertinent for the particular circumstances.

In clinical assessments, interprofessional relationships are critical for positive patient outcomes and continuity of care. The ability to recognize the strengths and weaknesses of your abilities is crucial to the team approach to patient assessment. Thoughts or suggestions from other medical professionals involved in the care of a particular patient or client can help the entire team successfully treat an individual. There are many areas of specialty in medical professions and it is prudent to seek out this expertise for the best patient outcomes. Interprofessional collaboration allows for the best use of all pertinent data to come up with the best care plan for a particular case.

The case studies in this workbook are designed to supplement medical nutrition therapy textbooks. These case studies may supplement a variety of nursing, pharmacy, and medical textbooks as well. Textbooks related to the assessment, intervention, and care of specific populations used by health professionals may serve as a good reference for those professions who choose to use this case study-based approach to interprofessional assessment. These case studies are designed to prompt critical thinking skills and determine several solutions to the same scenario. Furthermore, these case studies are designed to help novice practitioners proceed in a logical manner to address clinical concerns and serve as a tool to study for professional exams.

It is important to note that clinician guidance in interpreting these case studies in an educational setting is critical. There are many ways to evaluate the same sets of data. This is dependent on the background and primary professional focus of the learner and overseeing clinician. These case studies do not necessarily have one absolute correct answer as many methods of viewing the same case can be accurate. Discussing the different thought processes used to arrive at a particular assessment, intervention, or monitoring technique will enhance the development of critical thinking and patient assessment skills.

Recognizing the strengths of other health professionals and what they can contribute to the care in a particular case is critical in successful interprofessional healthcare team success and patient outcomes. The knowledge, strengths, and assessment skills of other team members will allow each individual team member to grow, develop evaluation and assessment techniques, and become a skilled interprofessional practitioner. These case studies are designed to address the benefits of working on interprofessional healthcare teams. Specific areas of each case study are meant to prompt the learner into investigating the additional insight and services that other team members possess to optimize patient assessments and interventions. Once the case studies are completed, the learner should be in a position to collaborate with members of any interprofessional healthcare team.

Learning Objectives

It is essential to have critical thinking skills when assessing any patient or client, especially the complicated ones. In the real world, it is rare to see an individual with only one particular problem or concern. Typically, patients or clients will have a variety of medical, social, economic, and educational concerns that need to be addressed for proper therapeutic intervention and outcomes. It may be unusual for one practitioner to be able to address all of the needs of a particular client or patient. Critical thinking skills allow each practitioner to evaluate data to determine what is pertinent for the particular case or scenario. Furthermore, these critical thinking skills will help to determine the best therapies for the patient or client as well as assist in determining what additional healthcare practitioners need to be involved so all of the patient's concerns can be properly addressed. Learning objectives for *Interprofessional Approach to Assessment from a Nutritional Perspective* include

Demonstrate critical thinking skills.

Recognize the importance of interprofessional relationships.

Promote interprofessional behavior and determine when referrals to additional healthcare professionals need to be made.

Identify roles and responsibilities of interprofessional healthcare team members.

Develop a strategy of interprofessional teamwork for addressing patient concerns and solving patient problems.

Prioritize data to determine what is most pertinent to address for the specific scenario or case.

Identify significance and deficiencies of various sets of data used to assess patients or clients.

Determine the need to obtain additional data for the completion of a thorough assessment and evaluation of the client or patient.

Predict possible side effects or complications that may arise in different clinical scenarios.

Diagnose malnutrition using the ASPEN/AND guidelines defining malnutrition.

Recognize limitations of malnutrition diagnostic criteria.

Interpret laboratory data.

Interpret indirect calorimetry data.

Identify drug–nutrient interactions.

Demonstrate the planning and use of therapeutic diets for specific conditions including DASH recommendations, Therapeutic Lifestyle Changes, CHO counting, National Dysphagia Diets, and the National Renal Diet.

Calculate and implement parenteral and enteral nutrition support therapy.

Identify goals for nutritional monitoring and evaluation based on the current needs of an individual.

Calculate fluid requirements and identify the need for changes in fluid intake.

Evaluate nutritional requirements and determine appropriate nutrition therapy when multiple medical and surgical concerns are present.

Evaluate ethnic variations of dietary modifications.

CHAPTER **1**

Patient Assessment, Therapeutic Interventions, and Addressing Malnutrition

When conducting a patient assessment and developing therapeutic recommendations, several items should be addressed to make sure that the best possible assessment and interventions are provided. Available data should be thoroughly investigated and appropriate referrals to additional members of the interprofessional health-care team should be made as needed. Addressing the patient's primary diagnosis and how this relates to the nutritional status and nutritional problems of the patient is critical to developing an appropriate nutritional intervention. Asking additional questions to fill in gaps in data or to clarify available data is important. One should not look at one piece of data to make assessments, but rather review trends in data to make a "better" nutritional assessment. Determining if the patient does or does not have malnutrition should be done in all patient assessments. The problems and costs associated with malnutrition are widely published. Once a nutritional assessment is made and nutritional problems are identified, a plan of action needs to be developed. This nutritional intervention needs to address all of the patient's nutritional problems. This intervention needs to be easy to follow and should be in a realistic approach to enhance patient success. Sometimes, the intervention must be completed in steps for better success. Overwhelming the patient with unrealistic goals will hinder success.

It can be a challenge to determine what needs to be addressed when assessing a particular patient or client. First, it is important to note that not all available data will be pertinent for a particular assessment to be completed. Critical thinking skills will enable the practitioner to determine what data are pertinent for the particular situation and what data can be used at a later date. Although all data are important, some of the data may not be important at the particular time of your assessment. It is also important to note that not all data are important to all practitioners. One piece of data can be useful in the overall assessment of a patient for all practitioners. Another piece of data may only be useful to one or two of the members of the health-care team.

The primary diagnosis is important to all members of the interprofessional health-care team involved in the care of a particular patient or client. This is the primary reason you are consulting on this patient and providing your expertise. Based on your area of expertise, the particular data available and the desired patient outcomes, you can prioritize the remaining data. Determining what data are critical in your evaluation of the patient, subsequent therapeutic recommendations and interventions should be top priority. Next, you determine what data are relevant to your overall evaluation and therapeutic recommendations, but not necessarily critical in achieving your desired outcomes for the patient. Finally, you determine what data may be useful to consider when making your evaluation and therapeutic recommendations, but could be of more use to additional members of the interprofessional health-care team. While this final set of data may not directly impact your assessment or intervention, it should not be discarded. This data may be useful when working on an interprofessional team; especially, if this data consists of information the patient verbally volunteered during an interview. If you uncover information that would assist another health-care team member in providing optimal care to the patient; it is your responsibility to make sure these data are documented and forwarded to the appropriate team member. If your team has weekly interprofessional patient care rounds or conferences, this would be a perfect forum to address many interprofessional issues. However, one should not wait until a scheduled conference to report pertinent information that can immediately impact patient care. Directly contacting the appropriate practitioner is always the best course of action. Let's say you are performing follow-up education on a diabetic patent. During your session, the patient cited that she no longer has a car to drive after her teenage child was in a car accident three weeks ago. The patient cited that she was relieved her child and no one else was hurt; however, since her child was at fault, this did cause a huge hardship in the loss of the vehicle that she cannot afford to replace. She also cited that she must now rely on her sister to take her to doctor's appointments, shopping, and to the pharmacy to purchase her diabetic medications. While this may not directly affect your diabetic education of this patient, it can indirectly cause concerns. Could someone else on the interprofessional health-care team provide resources or assistance for this patient? Relaying this patient and information to the health-care team social worker in a timely manner for support may provide the patient with a reasonable and economical solution to her problem.

Another important consideration in patient assessment is that each answer to a question or comment from the patient should lead the practitioner to another question to investigate. This can keep the practitioner on track with patient interviews. Questions to the patient will not jump around and the practitioner has a lower chance of forgetting to ask something important. If you are a Registered Dietitian Nutritionist (RDN) interviewing a patient and he cites the presence of a "cow's milk allergy," this should lead you to ask a few more questions related to this milk "allergy." You may ask if this is a diagnosed allergy or lactose intolerance. Are adverse symptoms seen only with the consumption of cow's milk or all cows' milk containing foods and beverages? Are milk alternatives such as soy or almond milk consumed in place of milk? Are these milk alternatives tolerated without adverse effects? These additional questions can help to clarify the specific circumstances related to the "cow's milk allergy" so a correct dietary intervention may be provided.

When reviewing data in any assessment of a patient or client, it is extremely important to evaluate the trend in the data. Determining if the data are stable, improving or worsening is critical in determining a course of action and interventions. In some cases, stable data are desired. If you are evaluating weight status in an elderly patient who recently finished successful chemotherapy and her weight is within normal standards and stable, no further intervention related to weight change is needed. This stable, normal weight is a desired goal for this patient. In other cases, stable data may not be desired so an intervention to make a change would benefit the patient. If you are evaluating an obese, elderly, type 2 diabetic patient who would benefit from weight loss and his weight has remained stable, additional intervention is needed to produce weight loss. Increasing or decreasing trends in data may be a desired outcome in specific circumstances as well. Increasing average morning fasting blood glucose levels in this obese, elderly, type 2 diabetic patient would warrant intervention as the trends are moving in the wrong direction. In this same patient, fasting morning blood glucose levels decreasing toward desired normal range levels would be ideal and no further intervention is needed. Each trend may be assessed as positive or negative depending on the particular circumstances.

Following are areas that could prove to be important in any nutritional assessment. Based on the primary problem or concern of your patient and your desired outcomes, these data can be prioritized to determine the best overall course of action and interventions to achieve the best outcome for your patient. While the following list is extensive, not all of the items on the list are pertinent to each patient or client. There may be additional items which are not listed that can be important to address as well.

1. Primary diagnosis, problem, or concern

2. Secondary diagnosis, problem, or concern. This may be included in the patient's medical or surgical history and could be relatively recent or an issue that has lasted for years.

   Example: Your patient had a cholecystectomy three years ago and must follow a low fat diet to alleviate adverse gastrointestinal symptoms.

3. Nutritional intake history. This includes many subsets of information:

   a. Energy, protein, fluid, and micronutrient intake from all sources

   b. Usual or typical intake including eating schedule, including nutritional support, and/or oral supplement schedule

   c. Consumption of oral nutritional supplements; including protein shakes, smoothies, and commercial nutritional supplements.

   d. Recent altered eating habits, either intentional or unintentional

   e. Food preferences and aversions

   f. Food patterns, jags, or beliefs; including disordered eating

   g. Prior dietary education, comprehension, and compliance

   h. Difficulties with chewing or swallowing; including dental and oral health (edentulous, xerostomia, etc.)

   i. Gastrointestinal issues affecting oral intake; including constipation, diarrhea, gastro-esophageal reflux disease (GERD), and anorexia.

   j. Difficulties with shopping or food preparation

   k. Food insecurity

4. Anthropometric data; current and historical including comparison to published standards

   a. Height/length and weight, BMI

   b. Body composition data; including bioimpedance analysis (BIA), dual-energy X-ray absorptiometry (DEXA), and computed tomography (CT).

   c. Presence of amputations or paralysis

   d. Percentage of weight change or loss over time

   e. Derived parameters including arm muscle area (AMA) or mid-arm circumference (MAC)

   f. Assessment of function including hand grip strength

5. Nutrition focused physical assessment data
   a. Skin, mucous membranes
   b. Muscle mass
   c. Fat stores
   d. Hair, fingernails and eyes

6. Laboratory and additional clinical data; including current and historical data. Evaluation of trends in laboratory data is critical for accurate assessments. Laboratory data can give a wealth of information regarding organ function, disease status, nutritional status, and deficiencies.
   a. Analysis of blood
   b. Analysis of urine
   c. Analysis of specific tissue biopsies
   d. Results of X-ray, CT, magnetic resonance imaging (MRI), or other imaging tests

7. Medications
   a. Prescribed
   b. Common over-the-counter products like acetaminophen.
   c. Herbs and alternative medications
   d. Vitamins and additional micronutrients, minerals, or trace elements

8. Educational, lifestyle, and personal influences
   a. Educational background and ability to understand health-related education
   b. Socio-economic status. Will the patient or client require supplemental services to obtain needed health-related interventions; example Supplemental Nutrition Assistance Program (SNAP), medication assistance, and/or transportation
   c. Ability to perform activities of daily living (ADL); food preparation, shopping, bathing, and dressing.
   d. Living environment. Does the patient live alone, with a spouse, adult children, a group environment, or a senior living facility?
   e. Overall well-being. Does the patient have social ties, pets; do they participate in regular activities; is the patient alone or withdrawn?

When performing a nutritional assessment on a patient, it is imperative that malnutrition be diagnosed in those who meet the criteria. Many published studies note the incidence of malnutrition among specific populations is high; specifically, the elderly, hospitalized patients and those with chronic conditions. Malnutrition is associated with an increased hospital length of stay (LOS), increased cost in the overall care of the patient, and increased morbidity and mortality. Nutritional repletion is a primary goal in malnourished individuals. It is important to note that not all thin individuals are malnourished. An obese individual can be diagnosed with malnutrition. Diagnosing malnutrition is a nutritional priority.

It is also important to note the actual disease or condition a patient has may have contributed to the patient's malnutrition. Knowing how this disease or condition affected the patient and caused malnutrition is important. "Fixing" the disease is not necessarily the primary concern of the practitioner involved in the nutritional care of the patient. "Fixing" the malnutrition is a primary concern. Nutritional repletion can help to improve patient outcomes. Once nutritional repletion has started, the patient may be better able to tolerate the treatment of the disease or condition. Examples of the effects of treatment include adverse medication effects, disease effects on the body, additional surgical procedures needed, or a feeling of anorexia or early satiety. Better outcomes are possible with better tolerance to the treatment of the disease or condition. Let's say we have an emaciated patient with emphysema. He has lost weight, has a poor oral intake, and has lost muscle and fat mass, therefore he will meet the American Society of Parenteral and Enteral Nutrition and the Academy of Nutrition and Dietetics (ASPEN/AND) criteria for a diagnosis of malnutrition. When performing his nutritional assessment and developing his nutritional care plan, the malnutrition should be a primary focus. The actual disease or condition that caused the malnutrition is a concern; however, this can be addressed in a somewhat different manner. The patient's specific disease symptoms and medication side effects that affect nutritional status are specific to the patient's care and should be addressed to help nutritionally replete the patient. The primary concern remains the malnutrition and how to reverse this process.

In the appendix of this workbook, you will find a worksheet to help determine what is important to address in the particular assessment you are performing, what can be addressed later, and what should be referred to another member of the interprofessional health-care team. After evaluating the problems and nutritional goals of your patient, a determination to assess for the presence or absence of malnutrition should be completed. It is important to note that there are published guidelines to determine the presence of malnutrition. This worksheet can assist in determining if an individual who may not yet have a defined case of malnutrition can develop malnutrition in the future.

Once you have determined the problems that need to be addressed and assess your client's concerns, you will need to develop an intervention plan that meets the needs of the patient. This nutritional intervention can be as simple as recommending the patient to consume an oral high-protein nutritional supplement twice daily between meals. The intervention can become very detailed and complex in many cases; especially, in patients who have multiple concerns that need to be addressed. Patients often do not present with just one problem, but may have a set of abnormal labs and a medical, surgical, and psychological history that make planning successful nutrition intervention a challenge. At this point, it may be best to first prioritize and address the most critical concerns before addressing all of the patient's problems. If you have a patient with a poorly healing diabetic foot ulcer, it is best to address the nutritional needs that will promote wound healing before addressing the patients' noncompliance with her diabetic meal plan.

The nutritional intervention needs to be clearly stated so that all members of the interprofessional health-care team understand the precise recommendations and goals for the patient. It must address all of the current nutritional priorities of the patient. One must also be forward thinking when making recommendations. The recommendations need to be realistic for the particular patient and scenario. It would be unrealistic to recommend to a cancer patient who has just finished a round of chemotherapy and lost 3% of his body weight in the last month to start eating 3,000 kcal/day to promote weight gain. Weight maintenance may be the initial goal for this patient; weight gain would be a future goal.

When citing nutritional goals, it is best to cite them in practical terms. If you assess a patient's energy goals and your calculations determine the patient requires 2,018 kcal/day, it would be unrealistic to expect the patient to consume exactly 2,018 kcal/day. Recommending the patient to consume approximately 2,000 kcal/day is realistic. Another example would be seen with volume recommendations. It is best to recommend volumes that are measured in a practical manner. One cup equals 240 mL of volume. If you determine your patient needs to consume an additional 227 mL of water every day, this is an unrealistic measure. It would be difficult for a patient to comply with this measurement due to the difficulty in measuring this exact volume. Furthermore, if the patient is in the hospital, it would be a challenge for nursing to guarantee that this exact volume was provided and orally consumed. Simply recommending an additional one cup or 240 mL water is appropriate. If your patient requires nutrition support or additional intravenous (IV) fluids you should make a practical recommendation. In general, for adult patients IV fluid, TPN or tube feeding rates are typically recommended in a unit of measure that ends in a 5 or 0. Therefore, it is appropriate to recommend rates at 50 mL/hr, 55 mL/hr, 60 mL/hr, and so on. If an hourly rate of 57 mL/hr is needed to meet a patient's needs, the clinician will either recommend rounding the rate up to 60 mL/hr or down to 55 mL/hr. This will make the "mental math" easier when calculating volume intake. The exception to this rule would be in the case of neonates, infants, small children, or in individuals that require a strict fluid restriction. In these circumstances, each milliliter of volume can make a difference.

Finally, your intervention must match your overall patient assessment. If you cite your patient needs between 55 and 70 g of protein each day, your recommendations should reflect this cited requirement. Your recommendations must provide an amount of protein somewhere in the 55–70 g/day range. It is ok to recommend an intake at the very top or bottom of the range. Once in a while, a RDN must recommend an intake outside of their assessed recommended ranges due to specific patient circumstances. Let's say you recommend a tube feeding that provides 45 g of protein/day and you cite the patient requires 55–70 g of protein/day. This is ok as long as you justify WHY you made a recommendation outside of your desired range.

Nutritional assessment and the development of appropriate interventions can be challenging. The continuously evolving condition of the patient and their data (labs, oral intake, etc.) will affect your assessments and recommendations. Over time, nutritional problems will resolve and new ones can develop. Frequent monitoring, reassessments, development of revised interventions, and follow-up are needed to ensure that the patient is on track for resolution of their nutritional problems.

REFERENCE LIST

Allard, Johane P., et al. "Malnutrition at Hospital Admission—Contributors and Effect on Length of Stay: A Prospective Cohort Study Form the Canadian Malnutrition Task Force." *Journal of Parenteral and Enteral Nutrition,* vol. 40, 2016, pp. 487–97.

Jensen, Gordon L., et al. "Nutrition Screening and Assessment." *ASPEN Adult Nutrition Support Core Curriculum*, edited by Charles M. Mueller, 2nd ed., American Society of Parenteral and Enteral Nutrition, 2012, pp. 155–69. Published in Silver Spring MD.

Malone, A., and Carol Hamilton. "The Academy of Nutrition and Dietetics/The American Society for Parenteral and Enteral Nutrition Consensus Malnutrition Characteristics: Application in Practice." *Nutrition in Clinical Practice,* vol. 28, 2013, pp. 639–50.

McClave, Stephen A., et al. "Guidelines for the Provision and Assessment of Nutrition Support Therapy in the Adult Critically Ill Patient: Society of Critical Care Medicine (SCCM) and American Society for Parenteral and Enteral Nutrition (A.S.P.E.N.)." *Journal of Parenteral and Enteral Nutrition,* vol. 40, 2016, pp. 159–211.

Nelms, Marcia, and Diane Habash. "Nutrition Assessment: Foundation of the Nutrition Care Process." *Nutrition Therapy and Pathophysiology*, edited by Marcia Nahikian-Nelms, 3rd ed., Wadsworth, Cengage Learning, 2016.

CHAPTER **2**

Importance of Interprofessional Relationships in Health Care

In today's health-care environment, it is not possible for one individual practitioner to address each issue or concern a patent may have. Medical care is complex, requiring expertise from multiple sources to provide optimal patient care. It is not possible or cost effective for one individual practitioner to research and manage each facet of a patient's needs. Pooling the expertise of multiple health-care practitioners; each with a specialized set of credentials, expertise, and services provide optimal cost-effective care. This pooling of professionals is accomplished with the development of an interprofessional health-care team. These teams may be small with only a handful of members working in a local endocrine clinic or can be large with over twenty members in a large teaching hospital's surgical or burn center. It is important that these individual practitioners work together to provide the best possible service and outcomes. Practitioners may have differences in opinions, but they need to be able to overcome these differences in a professional manner with the needs of the patient always coming first.

Part of being a successful member of an interprofessional health-care team is recognizing the roles and responsibilities of each team member. One must accept that the team works together to meet the needs of the patient. The patient is at the center of the team and meeting the patient's needs are the primary goal of the interprofessional team. Pooling resources from many health-care professionals often enable a team to effectively evaluate all aspects of the patient's condition and develop a plan to successfully meet the needs of the patient. It is important that all team members understand the educational background, typical services provided, and areas of specific expertise of each member of the team. This allows each member of the team to focus on the needs of the patient as they pertain to their areas of expertise. This allows members to defer decisions or recommendations for a particular problem to the team member(s) who are most qualified to make these decisions. Members who work together and recognize each team member's strengths will be able to function well as a group. One team member may look at a problem from a slightly different approach and the group conversations can then provide input or suggestions to come up with the best possible solution.

Ideally, the interprofessional team works together on all areas of patient care and always develops their plan of action based on what is best for the patient while considering the concerns of other team members. These teams provide patient-centered care. The teams may not necessarily meet daily, but should meet at scheduled times, possibly weekly to discuss individual patient's concerns from the perspective of each team member. Weekly patient care rounds can achieve this goal. Ideally, the weekly patient care rounds will take place in a conference room where all members of the interprofessional team can meet and discuss the patient while accessing the medical record so needed additional information can be quickly obtained. Patients and their history including current issues are introduced. Typically, a physician, physician assistant, or medical/surgical resident will present this information. During this team meeting, a list of medications is read, current laboratory values are presented, and any new or ongoing medical procedures are noted as well as the physician's goals for the patient. After the introduction, presentation of all current pertinent information and the primary physician's concerns are presented to the group. Each member of the interprofessional team will take their turn discussing their current concerns and recommendations for the patient. Members of the interprofessional team can also make suggestions to other team members when they are discussing their individual concerns. Each member of the team may also ask other members' thoughts and opinions regarding a particular patient concern.

To put this in perspective, let's say our interprofessional team is discussing a seven-year-old child that was in a car accident and suffered several fractured ribs and a femur fracture. The femur fracture required surgical debridement and repair. The child was riding in a car with his mother and grandmother who were also injured in the accident. The child is on an age appropriate regular diet. He is not eating well. The child is worried because he has not yet seen his grandmother since the accident which occurred ten days ago. His mother does come to visit him every evening. Due to the loss of transportation, the child's mother is now only able to visit him at the evening meal once her husband arrives home with their only car.

The orthopedic surgeon and pediatrician will lead the patient care rounds for this particular case. Typically, the pediatrician will manage the majority of patient needs and the orthopedic surgeon will manage the orthopedic injuries. The orthopedic surgeon notes that due to the extent of rib fractures, the child is expected to receive intravenous (IV) analgesics and remain hospitalized for two more weeks. The orthopedic surgeon notes that he is concerned about the child's low-albumin levels. The orthopedic surgeon wants to see an improvement in the patient's albumin levels before he goes back to the operating room for additional debridement of the injured leg. Nursing reports that the child is typically sleepy most of the day due to effects of multiple medications. The nurse also reports the boy cries frequently due to not being able to see his mother and grandmother during the day.

Several members of the interprofessional team can work with the dietitian when it is her turn to present her concerns regarding this patient's poor oral intake. The dietitian may suggest obtaining labs to help to determine if the patient is still actively in a stressful state. The dietitian can cite obtaining a C-reactive protein (CRP) and prealbumin will assist in the evaluation of the current albumin levels. If the CRP is high, the patient is still in an inflammatory state and it is unlikely that the albumin will rise. Furthermore, once the CRP starts to drop, due to a difference in half-lives, one will expect to see an improvement in the prealbumin well before one would expect to see an improvement in albumin.

The dietitian can ask the pharmacist if it is possible to alter the medications or medication schedule to allow the child to be more alert at mealtimes. The physical therapist will offer to get the child up in a chair versus lying in bed for mealtimes to try to enhance oral intake. The child life specialist may work on some distraction techniques at mealtimes to allow the child to focus on his meals rather than pain and his grandmother. The social worker may try to arrange for the child's grandmother, who is in the same hospital, to see the young boy. The social worker may also try to arrange for transportation so the mother can visit the boy during all mealtimes. The dietitian will discuss how she is working with the child to give him energy and protein dense foods he prefers to help with healing, growth, and development. All of these interventions by multiple members of the interprofessional team may help to enhance the boy's oral intake. Depending on how much the boy is actually eating and the nature of his lab values the dietitian may also suggest an oral pediatric multivitamin or nocturnal tube feeding.

Above is a perfect example of how the interprofessional team will work together to solve one problem of poor oral intake. Each member recognizes the dietitian is responsible for evaluating the nutritional intake and determining if it is adequate. Each team member also recognizes that they can pool their specific talents and areas of expertise to help the child achieve the dietitian's goal of adequate oral intake. The suggestions are all patient centered. The individual suggestions and contributions of each team member are valuable and appreciated.

Interprofessional teams may be large or small. The size of the team depends on the patient or client population and the needs of this group. An endocrinologist may have weekly patient care rounds with his office staff. This small team may consist of the endocrinologist, her physician assistant, a dietitian, and a nurse. A large hospital may have many interprofessional teams and many members on each team. Each floor, unit or wing may have a team. The nephrology physicians/unit will have a team. The oncologists may have two teams; one to discuss their inpatients and the other to discuss their outpatients. Team members will be assigned based on the needs of the overall patient group.

To thoroughly understand the scope of diverse backgrounds, area of specialty, and unique skills that each member of the interprofessional team can contribute to overall patient care, please note the educational background, professional training, roles and responsibilities of each team member as follows:

Primary Physician/Attending Physician (MD, DO)

Resident Physician in a Teaching Facility (MD, DO)

Physician Specialist (e.g., endocrinologist, cardiologist, orthopedic surgeon, psychiatrist, podiatrist, and physiotherapist)

Physician Assistant (PA)

Nurse Practitioner (FNP)

Registered Nurse (RN)

Certified Nursing Assistant (CNA)

Home Health Nurse (RN)

Registered Dietitian Nutritionist (RDN)

Clinical Pharmacist (Pharm D)

Registered Pharmacist (R Ph)

Physical Therapist (PT)

Occupational Therapist (OT)

Speech and Language Pathologist (SLP)

Respiratory Therapist (RT)

Clinical Psychologist (PsyD)

Social Worker (MSW)

Child Life Specialist (CCLS)

Recreation Therapist

Client Relations Advisor

Personal Care Assistant

REFERENCE LIST

Interprofessional Education Collaborative Expert Panel. *Core Competencies for Interprofessional Collaborative Practice: Report of an Expert Panel.* Washington, Interprofessional Education Collaborative, 2011.

Körner, Mirjam, et al. "Interprofessional Teamwork and Team Interventions in Chronic Care: A Systematic Review." *Journal of Interprofessional Care,* vol. 30, no. 1, 2016, pp. 15–28.

Josiah Macy Jr. Foundation. http://macyfoundation.org.

MacNaughton, Kate, et al. "Role Construction and Boundaries in Interprofessional Primary Health Care Teams: A Qualitative Study." *BMC Health Services Research,* vol. 13, no. 486, 2013, http://bmchealthservres.biomedcentral.com/articles/10.1186/1472-6963-13-486.

Wilk, Szymon, et al. "Using Semantic Components to Represent Dynamics of an Interdisciplinary Healthcare Team in a Multi-agent Decision Support System." *Journal of Medical Systems,* vol. 40, no. 2, 2016, pp. 1–12.

CHAPTER 3

Cardiac Concerns

- -

Case Study: Outpatient with Malnutrition and Heart Failure

Case-Specific Learning Objectives

- ✓ Identify the role of natural supplements in the promotion of health.
- ✓ Plan energy and nutrient dense nutrition therapy while considering additional dietary modifications in sodium and saturated fat.
- ✓ Evaluate ethnic variations of dietary modifications.

Our Patient: Sammy P. is a sixty-three-year-old retired respiratory therapist. He retired after experiencing a heart attack at age 58. He is of Asian descent, married, and has two children and three grandchildren. He started smoking when he was fifteen years old and quit ten years ago. Since retiring, Sammy has been very involved at the local community center. Due to Sammy's diminishing cardiac status over the past three years, he has decreased his trips to the community center and has had difficulty doing some activities of daily living like light yard work (raking leaves, pulling weeds, and trimming bushes) and washing his car. His twelve-year-old grandson now helps Sammy perform yard work and household repairs. Sammy has difficulty helping his wife vacuum the house or lifting heavy items.

Medical and Surgical History: Sammy experienced typical childhood illnesses. He has had hypertension and high cholesterol for the past ten years. He had hernia repair twelve years ago and suffered a myocardial infarction five years ago. Sammy was diagnosed with heart failure three years ago.

Home Medications: Sammy's daughter brings over a variety of over-the-counter natural products for him to take to improve his health. Sammy only takes these products a few times per week because he feels they do not help him. He currently has prickly pear cactus pad extract, coenzyme Q10, garlic extract, and grape seed extract in the house. His doctor has prescribed Captopril, metoprolol succinate, and bumetanide.

History of Current Illness: Sammy is being seen by his doctor for a routine three-month weight check and follow-up. He reports continued fatigue and difficulty with activities of daily living. Sammy cites that if he is on his feet for an extended period of time, his lower extremities become very swollen. Sometimes, Sammy is too tired to move from the chair in front of the TV and has been progressively having more Netflix binges. He still tries to help his wife around the house and help with some basic yardwork. Lately, Sammy reports that he acts more like a supervisor to his wife and grandson than an actual helper with these chores. Sammy reports that it has been difficult to eat much at mealtimes over the past six weeks. He tires easily when eating and does not feel like eating his meals or between meal snacks his wife prepares because they are "bland and lack flavor." Sammy's wife usually makes him half of a meat and veggie sandwich with fat and sodium free mayonnaise for a snack each after-noon. Sammy prefers a bacon, lettuce, and tomato sandwich with regular mayonnaise or a bowl of rice, edamame, and soy sauce for a snack; however, his wife will not allow this any-more. Sammy's biggest complaint is his food lacks flavor because his wife has modified her traditional recipes to comply with Sammy's low sodium and low saturated fat dietary modifi-cations. Due to the lack of flavor and Sammy's fatigue, he is too tired and unmotivated to eat more than a small portion of what is served.

Routine Three-Month Check-Up Doctor's Appointment

Height: 5 feet 6 inches; weight: 118 pounds

Weight three months ago: 124 pounds

Weight six months ago: 135 pounds

Weight one year ago: 140 pounds

Hand grip strength using dynamometer: Below average for age

Temperature, °F: 98.4

Blood pressure, mmHg: 135/85

Pulse, beats/minute: 85

Respirations: breaths/minute: 20

Pulse oximetry, %: 97

Physical Assessment: Sammy's doctor documented pitting edema, 2+ in bilateral lower extremities; general pallor; eyes with pale conjunctiva; deep hallowing of the tempora-lis muscle; protruding and prominent clavicle; prominent and visible scapula, and emaciated appearance.

Table 3.1: Quarterly Fasting BMP Obtained One Week Prior to Sammy's Check-Up.

Laboratory Values	Normal Ranges or Values	Sammy's Values	Sammy's Value (WNL, High or Low)	Implications or Assessment
Glucose, mg/dL	70–110	93		
BUN, mg/dL	10–20	14		
Creatinine, mg/dL	Male: 0.6–1.2	0.8		
Sodium mEq/L	136–145	142		
Chloride, mEq/L	98–106	101		
Potassium, mEq/L	3.5–5.0	4.7		
CO_2, mEq/L	23–30	27		
Osmolality, mOsm/Kg H_2O	285–295	278		

Table 3.2: Quarterly Fasting Selected CBC Values Obtained One Week Prior to Sammy's Check-Up.

Laboratory Values	Normal Ranges or Values	Sammy's Values	Sammy's Value (WNL, High or Low)	Implications or Assessment
Hemoglobin, g/dL	Male: 14–18	13		
Hematocrit, %	Males: 42–52	40		
WBC, SI units	5–10	6.4		
Red blood cell count (RBC), SI units	4.7–6.1	4.5		
Mean corpuscular volume (MCV), fL	80–95	79		
Mean corpuscular hemoglobin (MCH), pg	27–31	25		

Table 3.3: Quarterly Fasting Additional Labs Obtained One Week Prior to Sammy's Check-Up.

Laboratory Values	Normal Ranges or Values	Sammy's Values	Sammy's Value (WNL, High or Low)	Specific Implications or Assessment
Calcium, mg/dL	9.0–10.5	9.2		
Albumin, g/d	3.5–5.0	3.1		
Prealbumin, mg/dL	15–36	15		
Crp, mg/dL	<1.0	5.1		
HgbA1C, %	<6.0	5.4		
Transferrin, mg/dL	Male: 215–365	412		
Ferritin, ng/mL	Male: 12–300	15		
TIBC, mcg/dL	250–460	475		

Case Evaluation

Prioritize Problems and Identify Interprofessional Care

1. List in order of importance Sammy's medical/nutritional concerns.

2. Review the concerns listed in question 1. Specifically, which member of the health-care team should address each concern and how should the concern be addressed?

Disease Process and Laboratory Interpretation

3. Are there laboratory values or vital signs in the tables above that would be a concern regarding Sammy's condition? Explain.

4. Describe two to three chronic nutritional concerns that may be associated with heart failure. Describe how these concerns can lead to a diagnosis of malnutrition.

Anthropometric and Nutrition Assessment

5. What is your evaluation of Sammy's height/weight status at his most recent doctor's appointment?

6. What percentage of body weight has Sammy lost over the past three months? What is the nutritional significance of this weight loss?

7. What is the percentage of body weight has Sammy lost over the past six months? What is the nutritional significance of this weight loss?

8. a. At this appointment, can Sammy be diagnosed with malnutrition based on the ASPEN/AND guidelines? Explain.

    b. Are there specific nutrient deficiencies that Sammy's doctor can diagnose? Explain.

9. Calculate Sammy's total energy and protein requirements. Justify your reasoning for method to determine needs.

10. a. What is your general assessment of Sammy's overall nutritional intake prior to this most recent doctor's appointment?

    b. Can you determine if Sammy has been compliant with his low sodium and low saturated fat dietary modifications? Explain.

11. Can you determine if Sammy may have a diet deficient in energy, protein, or micronutrients based on his physical exam? Explain.

Medications

12. Describe the main function of each natural product provided by Sammy's daughter. Describe any possible adverse side effects or drug–nutrient interactions with these products.

13. Describe the main function of Captopril, metoprolol, and bumetanide. Describe any possible adverse side effects or drug–nutrient interactions with these medications.

Intervention or Recommendations

14. Based on Sammy's medical history and current status (weight, labs, etc.), what specific recommendations would you make to increase both the energy and protein content of Sammy's diet?

Monitoring and Evaluation: Patient Follow-Up

15. Please describe a desired nutritional care follow-up schedule for Sammy and specifically what should be addressed at follow-up appointments.

16. What specific dietary questions would you ask Sammy in a follow-up to see if he understands his prescribed diet?

Academy of Nutrition and Dietetics (AND) Medical Nutrition Therapy (MNT) Guidelines and Documentation for Dietitians

Nutritional Diagnosis Utilizing the PES Statements:

Nutrition Intervention and Goals Utilizing AND Terminology:

Nutrition Monitoring and Evaluation Utilizing AND Terminology:

REFERENCE LIST

American Heart Association, http://www.heart.org/.

Anne, Van Leeuwen, and Bladh Mickey Lynn. *Davis's Comprehensive Handbook of Laboratory and Diagnostic Tests with Nursing Implications*. 6th ed., F.A. Davis, 2015.

Boullata, Joseph I., et al. "Dietary Supplements." *ASPEN Adult Nutrition Support Core Curriculum*, edited by Charles M. Mueller, 2nd ed., American Society of Parenteral and Enteral Nutrition, 2012, pp. 313–27.

Charney, Pamela. "The Nutrition Care Process." *Pocket Guide to Nutrition Assessment*, edited by Pamela Charney and Ainsley Malone, 3rd ed., Academy of Nutrition and Dietetics, 2016, pp. 1–14.

Collier, Scott R., and Michael J. Landram. "Treatment of Prehypertension: Lifestyle and/or Medication." *Vascular Health and Risk Management*, vol. 8, 2012, pp. 613–19, https://www.ncbi.nlm.nih.gov/pmc/articles/PMC3502030/.

Jenson, Gordon L., et al. "Nutrition Screening and Assessment." *ASPEN Adult Nutrition Support Core Curriculum*, edited by Charles M. Mueller, 2nd ed., American Society of Parenteral and Enteral Nutrition, 2012, pp. 155–69.

Langley, G., and Sharla Tajchman. "Fluids, Electrolytes and Acid-Base Disorders." *ASPEN Adult Nutrition Support Core Curriculum*, edited by Charles M. Mueller, 2nd ed., American Society of Parenteral and Enteral Nutrition, 2012, pp. 98–120.

Malone, Ainsley, and Carol Hamilton. "The Academy of Nutrition and Dietetics/The American Society for Parenteral and Enteral Nutrition Consensus Malnutrition Characteristics: Application in Practice." *Nutrition in Clinical Practice*, vol. 28, no. 28, 2013, pp. 639–50.

Merck Manual Professional Version, http://www.merckmanuals.com/professional/nutritional-disorders/nutrition,-c-,-general-considerations/nutrient-drug-interactions.

Nelms, Marcia, and Diane Habash. "Nutrition Assessment: Foundation of the Nutrition Care Process." *Nutrition Therapy and Pathophysiology*, edited by Marcia Nahikian-Nelms, 3rd ed., Wadsworth, Cengage Learning, 2016.

Pagana, Kathleen Deska, and Timothy James Pagana. *Mosby's Manual of Diagnostic and Laboratory Tests*. Mosby/Elsevier, 2014.

Peterson, Sarah. "Nutrition Focused Physical Assessment." *Pocket Guide to Nutrition Assessment*, edited by Pamela Charney and Ainsley Malone, 3rd ed., Academy of Nutrition and Dietetics, 2016, pp. 76–102.

Pujol, Thomas, et al. "Diseases of the Cardiovascular System." *Nutrition Therapy and Pathophysiology*, edited by Marcia Nahikian-Nelms, 3rd ed., Wadsworth, Cengage Learning, 2016.

Case Study: Inpatient/Outpatient with Hypertension, Hyperlipidemia following a Myocardial Infarction

Case-Specific Learning Objectives

✓ Assess risk of developing additional complications from hypertension and hyperlipidemia.

✓ Plan appropriate intervention using the therapeutic lifestyle changes (TLC) principles.

Our Patient: Amy S. is a forty-eight-year-old accountant. She is employed with a large accounting firm in a large city and works eight to ten hour days each week. She is married and has two grown children in their mid-twenties. She takes public transportation into the city to work each day. This commute consists of walking half a mile each morning and afternoon. Amy stops by the market two to three days per week after work and carries her groceries on this half a mile walk. Amy loves to walk in the local parks on weekends and typically walks a few miles each weekend. Amy has a brother and sister who both have hypertension and high cholesterol. Her brother is three years older and had "artery bypass surgery in three veins" when he was fifty years old. Both of her parents passed away from "heart disease" when they were in their early seventies.

Medical and Surgical History: Amy suffered a broken right wrist when she was twelve. She had all of the typical childhood illnesses. Amy reports for annual check-ups each year and her blood pressure and lipid levels have been borderline upper limit normal for the past three years. She received brief education regarding lowering her salt and saturated fat intake three years agos. Due to Amy's strong family history of cardiovascular disease, she has been "fairly compliant" with this education. Amy does admit to some days where she cheats on her diet and exercise regime.

Home Medications: Amy started to take Lopressor to control her blood pressure and combination lovastatin–niacin to control her blood lipid levels three years ago.

History of Current Illness: Amy had just finished her shopping and was a block from her home when she started to feel lightheaded, nauseated, and dizzy. She was carrying one heavy bag of groceries and dropped it on the street. A college student stopped to help her. He noticed that Amy appeared uncomfortable and complained of chest, arm, and jaw pains. He immediately called 911 and the paramedics transported Amy to the local hospital.

Emergency Room (ER) and Day 1 Events: Amy presented to the ER in acute distress. Amy received sublingual nitroglycerine and oxygen. She received intravenous (IV) morphine to control her pain. Amy was transferred directly to the angiography suite where blockage of two major vessels was discovered. Amy received percutaneous coronary intervention (PCI) before being transferred to the cardiac care unit.

Anthropometrics

Height: 5 feet 3 inches; weight: 135 pounds

Body composition information: Unavailable

Laboratory Values and Pertinent Vital Signs

Amy's doctor ordered the following labs and vitals upon her arrival to the ER (nonfasting).

Table 3.4: Nonfasting BMP Obtained in the ER.

Laboratory Values	Normal Ranges or Values	Amy's Values	Amy's Value (WNL, High or Low)	Implications or Assessment
Glucose, mg/dL	70–110	165		
BUN, mg/dL	10–20	17		
Creatinine, mg/dL	Female: 0.5–1.1	0.8		
Sodium mEq/L	136–145	142		
Chloride, mEq/L	98–106	101		
Potassium, mEq/L	3.5–5.0	4.7		
CO_2, mEq/L	23–30	27		
Osmolality, mOsm/Kg H_2O	285–295	291		

Hospital Course: Amy remained in the hospital for a total of 2½ days. She had an uneventful stay in the cardiac care unit. She ate her "post-myocardial infraction (MI) cardiac progression" diet well. She took slow walks in the hallway when instructed to do so. Amy was interested in her in-hospital cardiac rehab education and was looking forward to participating in the outpatient cardiac rehab program at the hospital.

Discharge Medications: Amy received an angiotensin-converting-enzyme (ACE) inhibitor, beta-blocker, atorvastatin, and heparin in the hospital. She was discharged on the ACE inhibitor, beta-blocker, and atorvastatin. Her heparin was changed to Coumadin upon discharge.

Table 3.5: Non-Fasting Selected Additional Lab Values and Vital Signs Obtained in the ER.

Laboratory Values or Vital Signs	Normal Ranges or Values	Amy's Values	Amy's Value (WNL, High or Low)	Implications or Assessment
Hemoglobin, g/dL	Female: 12–16	15		
Hematocrit, %	Female: 37–47	39		
WBC, SI units	5–10	9.4		
Calcium, mg/dL	9.0–10.5	9.9		
Albumin, g/d	3.5–5.0	4.1		
Prealbumin, mg/dL	15–36	15		
Crp, mg/dL	<1.0	8.1		
HgbA1C, %	<6.0	5.2		
Cardiac troponins, ng/mL	<0.1	6.4		
Ischemia modified albumin, IU/mL	<85	127		
Temperature, °F	96.4–99.1	99.4		
Blood pressure, mmHg	Systolic <120 Diastolic <80	195/155, decreasing to 165/105 after nitrate administration in the ER		
Pulse, beats/ minute	60–100	105		
Respirations: breaths/minute	14–20	22		
Pulse oximetry, %	≤95	98		

Table 3.6: Fasting Lipid Panel on Hospital Day 2.

Laboratory Values	Normal Ranges or Values	Amy's Values	Amy's Value (WNL, High or Low)	Implications or Assessment
Triglycerides, mg/dL	Female: 35–135	288		
HDL, mg/dL	Female: >55	50		
LDL, mg/dL	60–180	215		
Total cholesterol, mg/dL	<200	265		

Rehabilitation Course: Amy was referred to an outpatient cardiac rehabilitation program which provided diet, exercise, and lifestyle changes Amy needed to make for long-term health benefits. Amy met with a Registered Dietitian Nutritionist for a comprehensive nutrition therapy plan. When reporting her typical dietary intake, Amy noted she ate everything YOU ate and had to drink yesterday :)

— —

Case Evaluation

Prioritize Problems and Identify Interprofessional Care

1. List in order of importance Amy's medical/nutritional concerns.

2. Review the concerns listed in question 1. Specifically, which member of the health-care team should address each concern and how should the concern be addressed?

Disease Process and Laboratory Interpretation

3. Describe the ATP III (American Treatment Panel) guidelines.

4. Are there laboratory values or vital signs above that would be a concern regarding Amy's condition upon admit to the hospital/ER?

5. Amy was at risk for having a MI. Describe her risk factors.

6. Does Amy meet the criteria for being diagnosed with metabolic syndrome? Explain why or why not.

7. Describe three chronic medical complications associated with hyperlipidemia.

8. Are the symptoms of a MI different for males and females? Describe the symptoms for both.

9. Describe the diagnostic testing Amy underwent to determine that she had a MI due to blockage of her major arteries.

10. Describe the PCI and coronary artery bypass graft surgery (CABG) procedures.

Anthropometric and Nutrition Assessment

11. What is your evaluation of Amy's current height/weight status?

12. Would you encourage Amy to lose weight at this time? Explain.

13. Upon admit to the hospital, can Amy be diagnosed with malnutrition based on the ASPEN/AND guidelines? Explain.

14. Calculate Amy's total energy and protein requirements. Justify your reasoning for method to determine needs.

15. What is your general assessment of Amy's dietary recall? Do you feel she is consuming adequate, excessive, or deficient energy and protein based on her nutritional requirements?

16. Can you determine if Amy may have a diet deficient in micronutrients based on her current typical dietary intake? Explain.

17. Can you determine if Amy may have been compliant with a low sodium and low saturated fat diet prior to her MI? Explain.

Medications

18. Describe the main functions of Lopressor and lovastatin–niacin. Describe any possible adverse side effects or drug–nutrient interactions with these medications.

19. Describe the main functions of ACE inhibitors, beta-blockers, and atorvastatin. Describe any possible adverse side effects or drug-nutrient interactions with these medications.

20. Amy was discharged on Coumadin. Describe the main function of Coumadin and any possible adverse side effect or drug–nutrient interactions.

Nutritional Intervention and Recommendations

21. What diet should Amy consume for the first twenty-four hours following her MI? For each food or beverage item/type, describe why this modification is needed.

22. A "post-MI cardiac progression" diet was ordered for Amy. Each facility may have a slightly different diet and progression. Describe the ideal "post-MI cardiac progression diet" that Amy will follow.

23. a. What are the Therapeutic Lifestyle Changes.

b. What are the unique properties of the diet components of the TLC and why are they prescribed?

    c. What are the unique properties of the lifestyle components of the TLC and why are they prescribed?

24. Amy's typical dietary intake consists of everything **YOU** had to eat and drink over the past twenty-four hours. Evaluate the foods from "Amy's" typical diet. Identify the foods that might not be acceptable for Amy to consume with her TLC changes. For each food identified as a potential problem, provide an appropriate substitute.

Food or Beverage Consumed	OK When Following TLC Modifications? Yes or No	If Unacceptable When Following TLC Modifications Make an Appropriate Substitute
Breakfast		
Lunch		
Dinner		— 3 oz baked salmon
		— 1/2 cup brown rice
		— 1 teaspoon olive oil
		— 1/2 cup black beans
		— 1 cup cooked brocolli
		— salad: 1/2 cup romaine lettuce, 1/2 cup spinach,
Daily snacks		1/4 cucumber, 1/4 cup carrots, 1/2 cup tomatoes, 1 teaspoon vinegar & olive oil dressing

Monitoring and Evaluation: Patient Follow-Up

25. Please describe a desired nutritional care follow-up schedule for Amy and specifically what should be addressed at follow-up appointments.

26. What specific dietary and lifestyle questions would you ask Amy in a follow-up to see if she understands the prescribed interventions?

27. Do you feel Amy will be compliant with her diet in the future? Explain.

Academy of Nutrition and Dietetics (AND) Medical Nutrition Therapy (MNT) Guidelines and Documentation for Dietitians

Nutritional Diagnosis Utilizing the PES Statements:

In hospital

In cardiac rehab program

Nutrition Intervention and Goals Utilizing AND Terminology:

In hospital

In cardiac rehab program

Nutrition Monitoring and Evaluation Utilizing AND Terminology:

In hospital

In Cardiac rehab program

REFERENCE LIST

American Heart Association, http://www.heart.org/.

Anne, Van Leeuwen, and Bladh Mickey Lynn. *Davis's Comprehensive Handbook of Laboratory and Diagnostic Tests with Nursing Implications.* 6th ed., F.A. Davis, 2015.

Charney, Pamela. "The Nutrition Care Process." *Pocket Guide to Nutrition Assessment,* edited by Pamela Charney and Ainsley Malone, 3rd ed., Academy of Nutrition and Dietetics, 2016, pp. 1–14.

Collier, Scott R., and Michael J. Landram. "Treatment of Prehypertension: Lifestyle and/or Medication." *Vascular Health and Risk Management,* vol. 8, 2012, pp. 613–19, https://www.ncbi.nlm.nih.gov/pmc/articles/PMC3502030/.

Jenson, Gordon L., et al. "Nutrition Screening and Assessment." *ASPEN Adult Nutrition Support Core Curriculum,* edited by Charles M. Mueller, 2nd ed., American Society of Parenteral and Enteral Nutrition, 2012, pp. 155–69.

Malone, Ainsley., and Carol Hamilton. "The Academy of Nutrition and Dietetics/The American Society for Parenteral and Enteral Nutrition Consensus Malnutrition Characteristics: Application in Practice." *Nutrition in Clinical Practice,* vol. 28, 2013, pp. 639–50.

Merck Manual Professional Version, http://www.merckmanuals.com/professional/nutritional-disorders/nutrition,-c-,-general-considerations/nutrient-drug-interactions.

Nelms, Marcia, and Diane Habash. "Nutrition Assessment: Foundation of the Nutrition Care Process." *Nutrition Therapy and Pathophysiology,* edited by Marcia Nahikian-Nelms, 3rd ed., Wadsworth, Cengage Learning, 2016.

NIH: National Heart, Lung and Blood Institute. ATP III at a Glance: Quick Desk Reference, http://www.nhlbi.nih.gov/health-pro/guidelines/current/cholesterol-guidelines/quick-desk-reference-html.

Pagana, Kathleen Deska, and Timothy James Pagana. *Mosby's Manual of Diagnostic and Laboratory Tests.* Mosby/Elsevier, 2014.

Peterson, Sarah. "Nutrition Focused Physical Assessment." *Pocket Guide to Nutrition Assessment,* edited by Pamela Charney and Ainsley Malone, 3rd ed., Academy of Nutrition and Dietetics, 2016, pp. 76–102.

Pujol, Thomas, et al. "Diseases of the Cardiovascular System." *Nutrition Therapy and Pathophysiology,* edited by Marcia Nahikian-Nelms, 3rd ed., Wadsworth, Cengage Learning, 2016.

Roberts, Susan. "Food and Nutrition Related History." *Pocket Guide to Nutrition Assessment,* edited by Pamela Charney and Ainsley Malone, 3rd ed., Academy of Nutrition and Dietetics, 2016, pp. 34–49.

CHAPTER **4**

Endocrine Concerns

- -

Case Study: Gestational Diabetes

Case-Specific Learning Objectives

- ✓ Plan an appropriate diet considering the presence pregnancy-associated glucose intolerance.
- ✓ Identify appropriate lifestyle modifications considering the presence of gestational diabetes.
- ✓ Evaluate ethnic variations of dietary modifications.

Our Patient: Sylvia D. is a thirty-three-year-old female of Hispanic descent. She comes from a large family and there is a strong family history of cardiovascular disease, type 2 diabetes, and gestational diabetes on both sides of Sylvia's immediate family. Sylvia is the oldest of four children and her mother developed gestational diabetes when she was pregnant with Sylvia. Glucose control returned to normal for Sylvia's mother approximately eight weeks after Sylvia's birth. Her mother was diagnosed with type 2 diabetes after the birth of her second child.

Sylvia and her husband own a successful Mexican restaurant which serves many authentic family recipes. Sylvia works part time managing the finances for the restaurant and is in the process of investigating the opening of a second restaurant on the other side of the city. Due to her family's medical history, Sylvia has promoted their restaurant as a "healthy alternative" to typical Mexican food. She has modified recipes to include more vegetables, legumes, and unsaturated fats. Sylvia started taking either yoga or exercise classes at the gym two years ago in anticipation of a planned pregnancy. She is aware of the complications associated with diabetes and wanted to try and minimize her risk of developing gestational diabetes. Sylvia does not smoke or drink alcohol.

Sylvia is currently in her fifth month of pregnancy. To date, her pregnancy has been uneventful. She recently took a routine oral glucose tolerance test (OGTT) and was diagnosed with gestational diabetes.

Medical and Surgical History: She suffered from typical childhood illnesses and had a mild case of asthma that required medications from the ages of eight to twelve. Sylvia has not needed asthma medication since the age of twelve. She has had no broken bones or surgical procedures.

Home Medications: Prenatal vitamins.

Typical Dietary Intake

Sylvia has been craving salsa since she became pregnant. She snacks on homemade low-fat tortilla chips and salsa during the day. Over the past four to five weeks, Sylvia has had a bowl of fried ice cream every afternoon before heading home from work. The fried ice cream is the only fried food Sylvia can tolerate; all other fried foods have been making her nauseous.

Breakfast: She likes tea, pastries, and fruits in the mornings. Occasionally, Sylvia will have eggs and fruited yogurt.

Lunch: Sylvia typically eats at the restaurant. She will usually have soup and/or salad for lunch. The salad will have either chicken, fish, and/or low fat legumes as a protein source.

Dinner: Sylvia cooks a big meal each evening for dinner. She will eat a wide variety of foods for her evening meal, but always adds her homemade salsa on top of everything she eats including potatoes, pasta, rice, vegetables, meats, and fish.

Follow-Up Appointment at Doctor's Office: Sylvia's doctor noted normal weight gain, fetal heart sounds, and uterine growth; abnormal glucose tolerance on OGTT performed one week ago.

Anthropometrics and Additional Data from Office Exam

Height: 5 feet 5 inches; current weight: 170 pounds; Pre-pregnancy weight: 145 pounds

Hand grip strength: Average for age

Chest and lungs: Clear, normal breath sounds via auscultation

Heart: Normal rate and rhythm

Eyes and mucous membranes appear moist

Temperature: 98.9°F

Blood pressure: 130/70 mmHg

Pulse, beats/minute: 95

Respirations: breaths/minute: 18

Pulse oximetry: 100%

Hannah Muise

Table 4.1: Sylvia's OGTT Results.

Laboratory Values	Normal Ranges or Values	Sylvia's Values	Sylvia's Value (WNL, High or Low)	Specific Implications or Assessment
Fasting glucose, mg/dL	<95	118	High	gestational diabetes
1-hour glucose, mg/dL	<180	205	High	gestational diabetes
2-hour glucose, mg/dL	<155	168	High	gestational diabetes
3-hour glucose, mg/dL	<140	154	High	gestational diabetes

Case Evaluation

Prioritize Problems and Identify Interprofessional Care

1. List in order of importance Sylvia's medical/nutritional concerns.

   1.) Diagnosed with gestational diabetes
   2.) strong family history of cardiovascular disease, type 2 diabetes, gestational diabetes
   3.) Consuming foods high in sugar, glucose, fat, carbohydrates

2. Review the concerns listed in question 1. Which member of the health-care team should address each concern and how should the concern be addressed?

   Sylvia should consult a doctor, dietitian, and diabetes educator regarding her diagnosis with gestational diabetes, nutritional intake, and family history. during pregnancy, affecting her glucose levels and blood sugar.

Disease Process and Laboratory Interpretation

3. What is gestational diabetes?

   Develops during pregnancy and affects how the cells use glucose. Can cause high blood sugar and increase patients risk of developing type 2 diabetes.

4. Describe complications associated with gestational diabetes?

   Causes high blood sugar which can affect the patients pregnancy and the baby's health. Gestational diabetes can cause a difficult birth, hypoglycemia in the baby, early preterm birth, excessive birth weight, and respiratory distress syndrome.

5. a. How is gestational diabetes diagnosed?

Diagnosed by using an oral Glucose Tolerance Test (OGTT)

b. Describe the OGTT test and expected results in someone with gestational diabetes.

1.) Initial glucose challenge test: drinking syrupy glucose solution. One hour later, blood test administered. Normal levels below 130 to 140 mg/dL. If higher, patient is at risk.
2.) Follow up glucose test: drinking higher concentration of glucose solution after fasting, blood sugar checked every hour, if 2 readings are higher than normal, diagnosis is given to patient

6. Does Sylvia have risk factors for developing gestational diabetes? Explain.

Her risk factors include that she has a strong family history of CVD, gestational diabetes and type 2 diabetes on both sides of her family.

7. Will the gestational diabetes be "cured" after Sylvia has her baby? Explain.

Sylvias blood sugar levels may go back to normal levels after delivery, but she poses a high risk of developing type 2 diabetes later in life.

8. What is Sylvia's risk for developing type 2 diabetes in the future? What is the risk of her baby developing glucose intolerance in the future? Explain.

Sylvias risk for developing type 2 diabetes in the future is high because she has gestational diabetes. Since there is a strong family history and genetic component, her baby has a high risk for developing glucose intolerance.

Anthropometric and Nutrition Assessment

9. What is your evaluation of Sylvia's pre-pregnancy height/weight status? Did this play a role in Sylvia developing gestational diabetes? Explain.

Sylvias pre pregnancy weight was slightly overweight for her height status. Depending on her fat mass compared to muscle mass her weight could have played a role in her developing diabetes.

10. Can Sylvia be diagnosed with malnutrition based on the ASPEN/AND guidelines? Explain. Sylvia has normal grip strength, normal breath sounds, normal blood pressure, and is not underweight. At this time, she would not be diagnosed with malnutrition. However, if she did not incorporate essential nutrients in her diet while having gestational diabetes, then she may run the risk of becoming malnourished

11. Determine Sylvia's total energy and protein requirements. Calculate these needs and justify your reasoning for method to determine needs.

EER: 354 - (6.91 × 33) + 1.27 (9.36 × U) + (7.26 × 1.05) + 340 = 2,772

Sylvia is fairly active and pregnant, so she needs an extra ≈300 calories per day. She should consume 2,772 calories per day, and 65 - 80 grams of protein for extra nutrients and energy for the baby.

12. What is your general assessment of Sylvia's typical dietary intake? Do you feel she is consuming adequate, excessive, or deficient energy and protein to promote a healthy pregnancy based on her nutritional requirements?

Sylvias typical dietary intake is fairly nutrient dense, except for eating fried ice cream and pastries everyday. To promote a healthy pregnancy, Sylvia should consume low glycemic index foods to lower her blood sugar, more protein and

13. Can you determine if Sylvia may have a diet deficient in micronutrients based on her current typical dietary intake? Explain.

omega-3 rich foods, more vegetables and whole grains, and limit fried foods, pastries, and excessive carbs and sugar.

Based on her typical dietary intake, it is difficult to determine if she has micronutrient deficiencys. She consumes a fairly healthy diet of fruits, vegetables, and protein and takes prenatal vitamins.

14. Can you determine if Sylvia may be consuming foods or beverages that may contribute to difficulties in controlling her blood sugar levels? Explain.

By consuming fried ice cream, pastries, fruit, potatoes, and salsa everyday, these foods may be contributing to Sylvias high blood sugar levels.

Medications

15. What diabetic medications would be unacceptable to use in pregnancy?

Any oral hypoglycemic agents are safe to consume during pregnancy. Other medications such as Thalomid, Accutane, and Claravis should be discontinued during pregnancy.

16. What diabetic medications would be acceptable to use in pregnancy?

Insulin, metformin, glyburide are safe and effective diabetic medications to use during pregnancy.

Nutrition Intervention and Recommendations

17. Describe appropriate diet therapy for Sylvia.

Sylvia should focus on a well balanced, wholesome diet of fruits, vegetables, legumes, lean meats, healthy fats, and some whole grains. She should follow a low glycemic index food diet plan and avoid foods that raise her blood sugar such as fried foods, pastries, and excessive amounts of sugar and carbohydrates.

18. Based on Sylvia's typical dietary intake, please develop a meal plan for Sylvia.

Food/Beverage and Recommended Time	Sample Meal Plan # 1 For Sylvia	Sample Meal Plan # 2 For Sylvia	Sample Meal Plan # 3 For Sylvia
Breakfast	• scrambled eggs • low fat plain yogurt with berries • whole ~~grain~~ wheat toast	• spinach & vegetable egg omlette with turkey bacon and tea	• buckwheat protein pancakes with strawberries and bacon
Midmorning snack	• handful of mixed nuts in yogurt	• blueberries in yogurt with cinnamon	• walnuts, pecans, almonds in yogurt
Lunch	• vegetable soup with spinach salad with chicken, added vegetables, olive oil, avocado	• tomato soup with crackers • turkey and cheese sandwich on whole wheat bread vinegar	• black beans with fish and sauteed vegetables • assorted vegetables with hummus and cheese slices
Midafternoon snack	• low fat plain yogurt with cinnamon and mixed nuts	• dried apricots or fruit low in sugar	
Dinner	• salmon with garden salad, olive oil and vinegar • black beans, vegetables, avocado with salsa	• shrimp with vegetables and spicy beans with salsa and avocado salsa	• grilled chicken with salsa and melted cheese • house salad with olive oil & vinegar
Evening snack	• dark chocolate in yogurt with no sugar dried fruit	• handful of walnuts, pecans, almonds	• dark chocolate in plain yogurt with blue berries

Monitoring and Evaluation: Patient Follow-Up

19. Please describe a desired nutritional care follow-up schedule and specifically what should be addressed at follow-up appointments.

She should follow up with a dietician for counseling and education on foods and meal plans that will promote a healthy pregnancy and lower her blood sugar levels. Diet, exercise, and medications should be addressed and glucose monitoring.

20. What specific questions would you ask Sylvia in a follow-up to determine if she under-stands her prescribed diet?
• What foods are you able to tolerate?
• Do you know what foods tend to spike your blood sugar levels?
• Do you understand what a low glycemic index food is?
• What nutrient dense substitutes can you make and tolerate to your current diet to promote low blood sugar?

Academy of Nutrition and Dietetics (AND) Medical Nutrition Therapy (MNT) Guidelines and Documentation for Dietitians

21. **Nutrition Diagnosis Utilizing the PES Statements:**
Inadequate energy, nutrient, and blood glucose levels related to high blood sugar and unhealthful diet as evidence by gestational diabetes diagnosis.

22. **Nutrition Intervention and Goals Utilizing AND Terminology:**
Carbohydrate modified diet for diabetes diagnosis, energy modified diet, protein and fat modified diet, general/healthful diet to promote healthful pregnancy with referral to RD in collaboration with doctor and pediatrician.

23. **Nutrition Monitoring and Evaluation Utilizing AND Terminology:**
Modified diet for diabetes diagnosis, avoidance of blood sugar rising foods and beverages, self monitoring and nutritional visits with RD, monitoring of blood glucose levels pre and post partum with RD and MD.

REFERENCE LIST

Academy of Nutrition and Dietetics. *Choose Your Foods: Food Lists for Diabetes.* Academy of Nutrition and Dietetics and American Diabetes Association, 2014.

American Diabetes Association, http://www.diabetes.org/.

_____. "Standards of Medical Care in Diabetes—2016." *Diabetes Care,* vol. 39, no. 1, 2016, pp. S1–S2, S1–S106, http://dx.doi.org/10.2337/dc16-S001.

Anne, Van Leeuwen, and Bladh Mickey Lynn. *Davis's Comprehensive Handbook of Laboratory and Diagnostic Tests with Nursing Implications.* 6th ed., F. A. Davis, 2015.

Charney, Pamela. "The Nutrition Care Process." *Pocket Guide to Nutrition Assessment,* edited by Pamela Charney and Ainsley Malone, 3rd ed., Academy of Nutrition and Dietetics, 2016, pp. 1–14.

Franz, Marian J., and Allison B. Evert. "Medical Nutrition Therapy for Diabetes Mellitus and Hypoglycemia of Nondiabetic Origin." *Krause's Food and the Nutrition Care Process*, edited by Kathleen Mahn and Janice L. Raymond, 14th ed., Elsevier, 2017.

Malone, Ainsley, and Carol Hamilton. "The Academy of Nutrition and Dietetics/The American Society for Parenteral and Enteral Nutrition Consensus Malnutrition Characteristics: Application in Practice." *Nutrition in Clinical Practice*, vol. 28, 2013, pp. 639–50.

Merck Manual Professional Version, http://www.merckmanuals.com/professional.

Nelms, Marcia Nahikian. "Diseases of the Endocrine System." *Nutrition Therapy and Pathophysiology*, edited by Marcia Nahikian-Nelms, 3rd ed., Wadsworth, Cengage Learning, 2016.

Nelms, Marcia, and Diane Habash. "Nutrition Assessment: Foundation of the Nutrition Care Process." *Nutrition Therapy and Pathophysiology*, edited by Marcia Nahikian-Nelms, 3rd ed., Wadsworth, Cengage Learning, 2016.

NIH National Library of Medicine Drug Information, https://www.nlm.nih.gov/medlineplus/druginfo/.

Pagana, Kathleen Deska, and Timothy James Pagana. *Mosby's Manual of Diagnostic and Laboratory Tests*. Mosby/Elsevier, 2014.

Roberts, Susan. "Food and Nutrition Related History." *Pocket Guide to Nutrition Assessment*, edited by Pamela Charney and Ainsley Malone, 3rd ed., Academy of Nutrition and Dietetics, 2016, pp. 34–49.

Case Study: Inpatient with Newly Diagnosed Type 1 Diabetes Mellitus Admitted with DKA

Case-Specific Learning Objectives

- ✓ Assess risk of developing complications associated with diabetes.
- ✓ Evaluate techniques for diagnosing type 1 diabetes.
- ✓ Interpret the symptoms of diabetic ketoacidosis (DKA).
- ✓ Plan an appropriate diet for an individual with type 1 diabetes using CHO counting principles.
- ✓ Understand the role and effects of insulin.

Our Patient: Hannah H. is a twenty-two-year-old flight attendant. She is single and lives with two roommates and their cats. On nights after an overnight trip she likes to go to happy hour, dance and have food and drinks with friends. She does not smoke or take illicit drugs. Hannah is fairly active, even when traveling. She visits the hotel gyms on overnight stays. She regularly participates in yoga or any fun class at her local gym when home.

Medical and Surgical History: Hannah considers herself to be healthy. She suffered from the typical childhood illnesses; colds, ear infections, and strep throat. She has never had stitches, or a broken bone but did suffer a sprained ankle two years ago when she tripped over her cat going down the stairs her home. She does have occasional outbreaks of psoriasis.

Home Medications: None.

History of Current Illness: For the past five weeks, Hannah has complained of fatigue, hunger, and thirst. She cites, she always seems to be eating or drinking water and her cravings are not satisfied. She reports frequent urination and her urine appears to have a different smell. She is concerned that despite eating more than usual she has lost weight; a total of 12 pounds in the last month. Last week, she stopped going to the gym because she was exhausted after work. She reports being too tired to go to the gym on her days off. This morning when she woke up, it felt like her heart was racing and she was hyperventilating. She had her roommate take her to the local emergency room (ER).

Emergency Room and Day 1 Events: Hannah presented to the ER around 9:00 a.m. She reported that she felt so bad and anxious that she did not eat breakfast before heading to the ER. She was drinking a bottle of water on arrival. Hannah reported that she was hungry and very thirsty. After a brief interview with the triage nurse and a finger stick to check blood glucose levels, the ER physician was notified that Hannah presented with symptoms of DKA; her accucheck only cited "high" and would not reveal an actual blood glucose level. Urinalysis showed ketones and glucose present. The ER physician ordered a ¼ normal saline (NS) IV to run at 75 mL/hr and bloodwork.

Anthropometrics: Height: 5 feet 6 inches; current weight: 123 pounds; weight four weeks ago: 135 pounds

Body composition information: Unavailable

Hand grip strength with dynamometer: Normal limits for age

Table 4.2: Fasting BMP Obtained in ER.

Laboratory Values	Normal Ranges or Values	Hannah's Values	Hannah's Value (WNL, High or Low)	Implications or Assessment
Glucose, mg/dL	70–110	674		
BUN, mg/dL	10–20	21		
Creatinine, mg/dL	Female: 0.5–1.1	1.1		
Sodium mEq/L	136–145	149		
Chloride, mEq/L	98–106	108		
Potassium, mEq/L	3.5–5.0	4.9		
CO_2, mEq/L	23–30	35		
Osmolality, mOsm/Kg H_2O	285–295	305		

Table 4.3: Hannah's ABG's in the Emergency Room.

Laboratory Values	Normal Ranges	Hannah's Laboratory Values in the ER	Hannah's Value (WNL, High or Low)	Implications or Assessment
pH	7.35–7.45	7.27		
PCO_2 mmHg	35–45	55		
HCO_3, mEq/L	21–28	30		
PO_2 mmHg	80–100	89		
O_2 Sat %	95–100	96		
Base excess, mEq/L	0 ± 2	−4		

Table 4.4: Fasting Selected Laboratory Data from CBC, CMP, and Additional Labs Plus Vital Signs Obtained in ER.

Laboratory Values or Vital Sign	Normal Ranges or Values	Hannah's Values	Hannah's Value (WNL, High or Low)	Implications or Assessment
Hemoglobin, g/dL	Female: 12–16	18		
Hematocrit, %	Female: 37–47	47		
WBC, SI units	5–10	8.8		
Albumin, g/d	3.5–5.0	4.3		
Phosphorus, mg/dL	3.0–4.5	4.0		
Beta-hydroxybuterate, mmol/L	<0.5	3.1		
C-Peptide, ng/mL	0.78–1.89	0.5		
Insulin autoantibody (IAA), units/mL	<0.4	0.8		
Islet cell autoantibodies (ICA), units/mL	<0.4	0.8		
Temperature, °F	96.4–99.1	99.6		
Blood pressure, mmHg	Systolic <130 Diastolic <85	145/90		
Pulse, beats/minute	60–100	110		
Respirations: breaths/minute	14–20	32		
Pulse oximetry, %	≤95	97		

Hannah was stabilized in the ER and given insulin. At 1:00 pm she was admitted to the medical intensive care unit (MICU) with a diagnosis of new onset type I diabetes mellitus (DM). The doctor wanted to keep her npo until her blood sugar values stabilized. She underwent frequent blood glucose checks and received insulin to control blood glucose levels while in the MICU.

Hospital Days 2 and 3: On hospital day 2, a CHO controlled breakfast was ordered . By the afternoon, Hannah's blood sugar values were ranging between 135 and 160 mg/dL with q 4 hour blood glucose checks. At this point, the endocrinologist ordered diabetic teaching from the Certified Diabetes Educator (CDE), RDN and a referral to outpatient diabetes "camp" that his staff runs in his office for all newly diagnosed diabetics.

On hospital day 3, Hannah was started on Lispro and Lantus in the morning. Hannah continued with the frequent blood glucose level checks; however, she rarely needed additional sliding scale regular insulin after the start of these new medications. She continued to receive her CHO-controlled diet and ate well; typically 90%–100% of each meal and evening snack. Blood glucose levels were checked before and after each meal as well as midmorning and before bed.

Hospital Day 4: Hannah was discharged directly from the MICU after receiving educational information over the past two days regarding diabetes, medications, and her diet. She was told by the Registered Dietitian Nutritionist (RDN), CDE that the information she received in the hospital consisted of survival skills and that she would receive comprehensive education at the outpatient diabetes camp. Her endocrinologist determined that Hannah needs approximately 30 kcal/kg and determined her discharge medication prescription should be 4.5 units of Lispro and 19 units of Lantus each morning. The endocrinologist also recommended that Hannah have an afternoon and evening snack each day, with each snack consisting of two carbohydrate servings at each snack (or a total of four servings for these snacks).

Typical Dietary Intake: When Hannah met with the RDN, CDE as an inpatient and again at the outpatient diabetes camp she reported the following typical intake. She always has a quick breakfast and it may vary depending if she spent the night in a hotel or at home. If she has breakfast at home she tends to eat more protein such as Greek yogurt, a boiled egg or toast, and nut butter. She always has coffee in the morning and prefers flavored sweetened coffee with cream. If Hannah is traveling, she will eat whatever is available at the hotel breakfast buffet, but tends to select more pastries and fruit with her coffee.

Lunch and dinner will vary as well depending on whether Hannah is traveling or not. If Hannah is traveling, she may have small frequent snacks and fewer meals during the day and will always have her evening meal with coworkers. Sometimes, this evening meal can be later in the evening; 8:00 or 9:00 p.m. If Hannah has a few days off, she is more likely to sit down and fix herself a; balanced lunch and dinner. She will eat these more at "typical meal times." Hannah denies food allergies, intolerances, or aversions. She will eat a wide variety of foods and there are no foods she will not eat or try. Hannah does report a sweet tooth and likes to have some small sweet item each night she is home; typically ice cream or a cookie. Hannah reports a dislike for milk, but she will drink it on occasion. She prefers to drink water or sweetened tea; iced or hot during the day and for her evening meal. She will have a couple of beers or cocktails when out dancing with friends.

Case Evaluation

Prioritize Problems and Identify Interprofessional Care

    1. List in order of importance Hannah's medical/nutritional concerns.

2. Review the concerns listed in question 1. Which member of the health-care team should address each concern and how should the concern be addressed?

Disease Process and Laboratory Interpretation

3. Are there any laboratory values or vital signs from Hannah's admit to the ER that would be a concern with regards to Hannah's condition?

4. Describe the symptoms that are associated with DKA. Did Hannah present to the ER with these symptoms?

5. Describe the laboratory changes that are present when someone develops DKA and why these changes occur. Did Hannah present to the ER with these lab changes?

6. Why did the ER physician fail to obtain Hannah's HgbA1C with the other labs?

7. The ER physician ordered a specific set of labs to assist in diagnosing Hannah with type 1 DM? What is the significance of each of the following labs?
   a. Beta-hydroxybuterate

   b. C-Peptide

   c. Insulin Autoantibody (IAA)

    d. Islet Cell Autoantibodies (ICA)

8. Describe three chronic medical complications associated with type 1 DM? Describe how chronic hyperglycemia promotes development of these complications.

Anthropometric and Nutrition Assessment

9. What is your evaluation of Hannah's height/weight status prior to the development of symptoms associated with type 1 DM?

10. What is your evaluation of Hannah's height/weight status upon presentation to the ER?

11. What was Hannah's percentage of weight change over the last four weeks? Are there concerns regarding this weight change? Explain.

12. Upon admit, can Hannah be diagnosed with malnutrition based on the ASPEN/AND guidelines? Explain.

13. Calculate Hannah's total energy and protein requirements. Justify your reasoning for method to determine needs.

14. What is your general assessment of Hannah's typical dietary intake? Do you feel she is consuming adequate, excessive, or deficient energy and protein based on her nutritional requirements?

15. Can you determine if Hannah may have a diet deficient in micronutrients based on her current typical dietary intake? Explain.

16. Based on this typical dietary intake do you think Hannah will have to make major changes to comply with the therapeutic changes needed to control her blood sugar in the future? Explain.

Medications

17. Could something other than insulin, example oral hypoglycemic agents be ordered for Hannah? Explain.

18. Why were both Lispro and Lantus ordered?

19. Can the Lispro and Lantus be mixed and administered with one syringe each morning? Explain.

20. Describe the onset, peak and duration of Lispro and Lantus.

21. Describe possible adverse side effects of drug-nutrient interactions with Lispro and Lantus.

Nutrition Intervention and Recommendations

22. Describe appropriate nutrition therapy for a person with type 1 DM.

23. How many grams of CHO are in each carbohydrate serving? Cite all food groups that contain approximately one CHO serving per portion?

24. **a.** Assuming Hannah is prescribed one unit of insulin per 10 g of CHO ingested at breakfast, how many grams of CHO should Hannah consume at breakfast?

    b. How many CHO servings does this equal?

25. Based on Hannah's energy, protein and CHO serving requirements, complete the following table to provide Hannah with a sample meal plan to follow. Include adequate CHO servings for each meal or snack to insure that Hannah receives adequate CHO for the insulin to act upon. Please use/modify the following table to map out Hannah's meal plan. For this exercise assume Hannah requires 10 grams of CHO for each unit of insulin prescribed.

Food and Beverage items	G CHO	CHO Servings	G Pro	G Fat	Kcal
EX. ½ cup applesauce	**15**	**1**	**0**	**0**	**60**
Breakfast Items (Need 3 CHO Servings)					
Lunch items (need ___ CHO servings)					
Afternoon snack (need ___ CHO servings)					
Dinner items(need ___ CHO servings)					

Food and Beverage items	G CHO	CHO Servings	G Pro	G Fat	Kcal
PM snack (need ___ CHO servings)					
Grand totals		___ total for the day			

Monitoring and Evaluation: Patient Follow-Up

26. Please describe a desired nutritional care follow-up schedule for Hannah and specifically what should be addressed at follow-up appointments.

27. What specific questions would you ask Hannah to make sure she understands her prescribed diet?

28. Do you feel Hannah will be compliant with her diet upon discharge? Explain.

Academy of Nutrition and Dietetics (AND) Medical Nutrition Therapy (MNT) Guidelines and Documentation for Dietitians

Nutrition Diagnosis Utilizing the PES Statements:
Inpatient

Outpatient

Nutrition Intervention and Goals Utilizing AND Terminology:
Inpatient

Outpatient

Nutrition Monitoring and Evaluation Utilizing AND Terminology:
Inpatient

Outpatient

REFERENCE LIST

American Diabetes Association, http://www.diabetes.org/.

_____. "Standards of Medical Care in Diabetes 2016." *Diabetes Care,* vol. 39, no. 1, 2016, pp. S1–S2, http://dx.doi.org/10.2337/dc16-S001.

Anne, Van Leeuwen, and Bladh Mickey Lynn. *Davis's Comprehensive Handbook of Laboratory and Diagnostic Tests with Nursing Implications.* 6th ed., F. A. Davis, 2015.

Ayers, Phil, et al. "Acid-Base Disorders: Learning the Basics." *Nutrition in Clinical Practice,* vol. 30, 2015, pp. 14–20.

Choose Your Foods: Food Lists for Diabetes. Academy of Nutrition and Dietetics and American Diabetes Association, 2014.

Charney, Pamela. "The Nutrition Care Process." *Pocket Guide to Nutrition Assessment,* edited by Pamela Charney and Ainsley Malone, 3rd ed., Academy of Nutrition and Dietetics, 2016, pp. 1–14.

Franz, Marian J, and Allison B. Evert. "Medical Nutrition Therapy for Diabetes Mellitus and Hypoglycemia of Nondiabetic Origin." *Krause's Food and the Nutrition Care Process,* edited by Kathleen Mahn and Janice L. Raymond, 14th ed., Elsevier, 2017.

Langley, G., and S. Tajchman. "Fluids, Electrolytes and Acid-Base Disorders." *ASPEN Adult Nutrition Support Core Curriculum,* edited by Charles M. Mueller, 2nd ed., American Society of Parenteral and Enteral Nutrition, 2012, pp. 98–120.

Malone, Ainsley, and Carol Hamilton. "The Academy of Nutrition and Dietetics/The American Society for Parenteral and Enteral Nutrition Consensus Malnutrition Characteristics: Application in Practice." *Nutrition in Clinical Practice,* vol. 28, 2013, pp. 639–50.

Merck Manual Professional Version, http://www.merckmanuals.com/professional/.

Nelms, Marcia Nahikian. "Diseases of the Endocrine System." *Nutrition Therapy and Pathophysiology,* edited by Marcia Nahikian-Nelms, 3rd ed.,Wadsworth, Cengage Learning, 2016.

Nelms, Marcia, and Diane Habash. "Nutrition Assessment: Foundation of the Nutrition Care Process." *Nutrition Therapy and Pathophysiology,* edited by Marcia Nahikian-Nelms, 3rd ed., Wadsworth, Cengage Learning, 2016.

Newton, Laura, and Timothy Garvey. "Nutritional and Medical Management of Diabetes Mellitus in Hospitalized Patients." *ASPEN Adult Nutrition Support Core Curriculum,* edited by Charles Mueller, 2nd ed., American Society of Parenteral and Enteral Nutrition, 2012, pp. 580–602.

Pagana, Kathleen Deska, and Timothy James Pagana. *Mosby's Manual of Diagnostic and Laboratory Tests.* Mosby/Elsevier, 2014.

Peterson, Sarah J. "Nutrition Focused Physical Assessment." *Pocket Guide to Nutrition Assessment,* edited by Pamela Charney and Ainsley Malone, 3rd ed., Academy of Nutrition and Dietetics, 2016, pp. 76–102.

Roberts, S. "Food and Nutrition Related History." *Pocket Guide to Nutrition Assessment,* edited by Pamela Charney and Ainsley Malone, 3rd ed., Academy of Nutrition and Dietetics, 2016, pp. 34–49.

Case Study: Outpatient Diagnosed with Type 2 Diabetes Mellitus Requiring Insulin

Case-Specific Learning Objectives

- ✓ Assess risk of developing complications associated with diabetes.
- ✓ Evaluate techniques for diagnosing type 2 diabetes.
- ✓ Plan an appropriate diet for an individual with type 2 diabetes.
- ✓ Understand the role and effects or oral hypoglycemic medications.

Our Patient: Rick S. is a forty-five-year-old architect. He is married and has a twelve-year-old son and a fourteen-year-old daughter. Rick's wife is a nurse and works at the local elementary school. Rick owns his business and typically works ten hours per day. He does like to jog each morning and coaches his son's soccer team three nights per week. He does not smoke or take illicit drugs.

Medical and Surgical History: Rick was very athletic when he was younger. He played soccer and basketball until he was in eighth grade. He suffered a broken right radius and ulna after falling off his skateboard when he was eight. He broke three fingers playing basketball in junior high and tore his left rotator cuff during a football game during his junior year of high school. The shoulder injury in high school required surgical repair.

Four years ago, Rick went in for a routine check-up at the urging of his wife. He had not received a physical exam in several years. She noticed Rick was gaining weight, he complained of blurred vision, and easily becoming fatigued. Both of Rick's parents and his older brother have type 2 diabetes mellitus (DM). Rick was diagnosed with type 2 DM after blood work ordered at this appointment was performed. At the time of diagnosis, Rick's Hgb A1C was 9.4% and his weight was 235 pounds. Rick was placed on oral diabetic medications. He received education regarding blood glucose monitoring, diet modifications to promote weight loss, and overall care to minimize the risk of complications for the diabetic patient. Rick expressed concern for long-term complications with this diagnosis.

Home Medications: Rick has been taking Metformin and Glipizide daily since the diagnosis of type 2 DM. Medication doses have been adjusted over the past four years to control Rick's blood glucose levels.

History of Current Illness: Again at the urging of his wife, Rick scheduled a comprehensive follow-up appointment with his doctor. He has been having a difficult time controlling his blood glucose levels each day. His fasting morning blood glucose levels range from 180 to 200 mg/dL and his accuchecks during the day are running between 175 and 195 mg/dL. He reports feeling fatigued by the end of each day. He cites compliance with his diet, medication, and exercise regime.

Anthropometrics in the Doctor's Office

Height: 6 feet 0 inches; current weight: 205 pounds; weight four years ago: 235 pounds

Waist measurement: 42 inches

Body composition information: Unavailable

Hand grip strength with dynamometer: Normal limits for age

Temperature: 98.6°F

Blood pressure: 125/80 mmHg

Pulse: 75 beats/minute

Oxygen saturation: 99%

Table 4.5: Fasting BMP and Osmolality Obtained Four Days Before Scheduled Appointment

Laboratory Values	Normal Ranges or Values	Rick's Values	Rick's Value (WNL, High or Low)	Implications or Assessment
Glucose, mg/dL	70–110	188		
BUN, mg/dL	10–20	15		
Creatitnine, mg/dL	Male: 0.6–1.2	1.0		
Sodium, mEq/L	136–145	142		
Chloride, mEq/L	98–106	102		
Potassium. mEq/L	3.5–5.0	4.7		
CO_2, mmol/L	23–30	28		
Osmolality, mOsm/Kg H_2O	285–295	292		

Typical Dietary Intake

Breakfast: A quick meal consisting of coffee with creamer and sugar; Greek yogurt and granola or a bagel and a piece of fresh fruit.

Lunch at work: Some type of deli take-out meal is delivered to Rick at the office. He usually has a large meat sandwich (turkey or roast beef with cheese and veggies) and either a cup of hearty soup or a salad (pasta, three bean, cole slaw, or potato). He will snack on either fresh or dried fruit and a few handfuls of nuts during the day. Rick cites his lunch serving sizes as "typical take-out portions."

Dinner at home: Baked or grilled meat: usually chicken, steak, or fish plus potatoes; rice or pasta; a dinner roll or piece of whole grain bread with butter and a large mixed veggie salad with assorted dressings. Rick only occasionally has alcohol since his diagnosis; he will have a glass or wine or beer with dinner a couple nights a month. Rick cites his dinner serving sizes as "large." Rick drinks a lot of iced tea during the day and switches to water when he arrives home from work.

Physician Recommendations: Rick's physician was pleased with his overall weight and compliance to his medical therapies. His physician was concerned about Rick's overall increasing fasting and postprandial blood glucose levels. He determined that Rick would benefit from insulin therapy and ordered 6 units of Lispro and 10 units of Lantus to be administered each morning in addition to Rick's previous medications.

— —

Case Evaluation

Prioritize Problems and Identify Interprofessional Care

1. List in order of importance Rick's medical/nutritional concerns.

2. Review the concerns listed in question 1. Which member of the health-care team should address each concern and how should the concern be addressed?

Disease Process and Laboratory Interpretation

3. Are there any laboratory values or vital signs above that would be a concern with regards to Rick's current condition?

4. What was the significance of Rick's HgbA1C when labs were obtained four days prior to his doctor's appointment?

5. What is the significance of Rick's current morning fasting blood glucose results?

6. Rick was diagnosed with type 2 diabetes four years ago. Describe how this is typically diagnosed.

7. Rick may be at risk for developing some acute complications associated with type 2 DM. Describe the following acute diabetic complications and Rick's current risk of developing each complication.
   a. DKA

   b. Dawn phenomenon

   c. Hyperosmolar hyperglycemic state (HHS)

8. a. Describe metabolic syndrome. Does Rick meet criteria to be currently diagnosed with metabolic syndrome?

   b. What would have to change for Rick to be diagnosed with metabolic syndrome in the future?

9. Describe three chronic medical complications associated with DM? Describe how chronic hyperglycemia promotes the development of these complications.

Anthropometric and Nutrition Assessment

10. What is your evaluation of Rick's current height/weight status?

11. What is Rick's percentage of weight change over the last four years? Are there any concerns regarding this weight change? Explain.

12. Would you encourage Rick to lose more weight at this time? Explain.

13. Can Rick be diagnosed with malnutrition based on the ASPEN/AND guidelines? Explain.

14. Calculate Rick's total energy and protein requirements. Justify your reasoning for method to determine needs.

15. What is your general assessment of Rick's typical dietary intake? Do you feel he is consuming adequate, excessive, or deficient energy and protein based on his nutritional requirements?

16. Can you determine if Rick may have a diet deficient in micronutrients based on his current typical dietary intake? Explain.

Medications

17. Describe the main function of Metformin and Glipizide. Describe any possible adverse side effects or drug–nutrient interactions with these medications.

18. a. Describe the insulin therapy that was started for Rick. Why did Rick have to start insulin?

b. Describe the onset, peak and duration of action for both Lispro and Lantus.

19. Rick will continue to receive his Metformin and Glipizide in addition to insulin. Does this mean that his pancreas is still producing some insulin? Explain.

Nutrition Intervention and Recommendations

20. Describe appropriate nutrition therapy for a person with type 2 DM.

21. How must Rick's diet change once insulin therapy is initiated?

22. How many grams of CHO are in each carbohydrate serving? Cite all food groups that contain approximately one CHO serving per portion?

23. a. Assuming Rick is prescribed one unit of insulin per 10 g of CHO ingested at breakfast, how many grams of CHO should Rick consume at breakfast? Note: this question only considers exogenous insulin administration.

b. How many CHO servings does this equal?

24. Based on Rick's energy and protein requirements, revise his diet to prevent overconsumption of energy (if present) and adequate protein. Include CHO servings for each meal to insure that Rick understands CHO servings in light of the receipt of some insulin each day. Make sure adequate CHO is provided for breakfast. Please use/modify the following table to map out Rick's meal plan. Remember Rick is receiving oral hypoglycemic agents so insulin will not cover all CHO ingested.

Food or Beverage items	G CHO	CHO Servings	G Pro	G Fat	Kcal
EX. ½ cup applesauce	**15**	**1**	**0**	**0**	**60**
Breakfast Items					
Lunch items					
Dinner items					
PM snack					
Grand totals					

Monitoring and Evaluation: Patient Follow-Up

25. Please describe a desired nutritional care follow-up schedule for Rick and specifically what should be addressed at follow-up appointments.

26. What specific questions would you ask Rick to make sure he understands his prescribed diet?

Academy of Nutrition and Dietetics (AND) Medical Nutrition Therapy (MNT) Guidelines and Documentation for Dietitians

Nutrition Diagnosis Utilizing the PES Statements:

Nutrition Intervention and Goals Utilizing AND Terminology:

Nutrition Monitoring and Evaluation Utilizing AND Terminology:

REFERENCE LIST

[REFS]Academy of Nutrition and Dietetics. *Choose Your Foods: Food Lists for Diabetes.* Academy of Nutrition and Dietetics and American Diabetes Association, 2014.

American Diabetes Association, http://www.diabetes.org/.

_____. "Standards of Medical Care in Diabetes 2016." *Diabetes Care,* vol. 39, no. 1, 2016, pp. S1–S2, http://dx.doi.org/10.2337/dc16-S001.

Anne, Van Leeuwen, and Bladh Mickey Lynn. *Davis's Comprehensive Handbook of Laboratory and Diagnostic Tests with Nursing Implications.* 6th ed., F. A. Davis, 2015.

Charney, Pamela. "The Nutrition Care Process." *Pocket Guide to Nutrition Assessment*, edited by Pamela Charney and Ainsley Malone, 3rd ed., Academy of Nutrition and Dietetics, 2016, pp. 1–14.

Malone, Ainsley, and Carol Hamilton. "The Academy of Nutrition and Dietetics / The American Society for Parenteral and Enteral Nutrition Consensus Malnutrition Characteristics: Application in Practice." *Nutrition in Clinical Practice,* vol. 28, 2013, pp. 639–50.

Marian, J. Franz, and Allison B. Evert. "Medical Nutrition Therapy for Diabetes Mellitus and Hypoglycemia of Nondiabetic Origin." *Krause's Food and the Nutrition Care Process*, edited by Kathleen Mahn and Janice L. Raymond, 14th ed., Elsevier, 2017.

Merck Manual Professional Version, http://www.merckmanuals.com/professional/.

Nelms, Marcia Nahikian. "Diseases of the Endocrine System." *Nutrition Therapy and Pathophysiology*, edited by Marcia Nahikian-Nelms, 3rd ed., Wadsworth, Cengage Learning, 2016.

Nelms, Marcia, and Diane Habash. "Nutrition Assessment: Foundation of the Nutrition Care Process." *Nutrition Therapy and Pathophysiology*, edited by Marcia Nahikian-Nelms, 3rd ed., Wadsworth, Cengage Learning, 2016.

Newton, L., and Timothy Garvey. "Nutritional and Medical Management of Diabetes Mellitus in Hospitalized Patients." *ASPEN Adult Nutrition Support Core Curriculum*, edited by Charles Mueller, 2nd ed., American Society of Parenteral and Enteral Nutrition, 2012, pp. 580–602.

Pagana, Kathleen Deska, and Timothy James Pagana. *Mosby's Manual of Diagnostic and Laboratory Tests*. Mosby/Elsevier, 2014.

Peterson, Sarah J. "Nutrition Focused Physical Assessment." *Pocket Guide to Nutrition Assessment, edited by* Pamela Charney and Ainsley Malone, 3rd ed., Academy of Nutrition and Dietetics, 2016, pp. 76–102.

Roberts, S. "Food and Nutrition Related History." *Pocket Guide to Nutrition Assessment, edited by* Pamela Charney and Ainsley Malone, 3rd ed., Academy of Nutrition and Dietetics, 2016, pp. 34–49.

Case Study: Inpatient with Complications Including Type 2 Diabetes Mellitus, Metabolic Syndrome, and a Gangrenous Lower Extremity

Case-Specific Learning Objectives

- ✓ Assess nutritional requirements when considering the presence of additional complications associated with diabetes.
- ✓ Plan appropriate nutritional support therapy when considering the presence of additional complications associated with diabetes.
- ✓ Understand the effects of complications associated with type 2 diabetes.

Our Patient: Please refer to part 1 of this case to obtain additional pertinent personal, medical, surgical, dietary and medication history on Rick. It is now twenty years later.

Rick S. is a sixty-five-year-old architect. He is married and has two grown children and one grandchild. Rick's wife is a retired nurse. Rick owns his business and is in the process of turning the business over to his son who is also an architect. Rick now works approximately six hours per day. He used to be very active, but admits he has "slowed down" once he turned sixty. Rick and his wife like to walk 1–2 miles daily whenever the weather is nice. He does not smoke or take illicit drugs.

Medical and Surgical History: Rick was diagnosed with type 2 diabetes when he was forty-one years old. Overall he has been compliant with his medication and nutritional therapy. He took oral hypoglycemic agents for four years before advancing to taking insulin in addition to the oral agents. Rick's weight has fluctuated over the years; however, since he turned sixty, his weight has been slowly increasing. After being diagnosed with type 2 diabetes, Rick's lowest body weight was 190 pounds when he was forty-eight years old. Rick was diagnosed with metabolic syndrome four years ago. Over the past six months, he has reported diminished feeling in his feet.

Home Medications: Rick has been taking Metformin and Glipizide daily since the diagnosis of type 2 DM. Rick takes Lantus and Lispro every day as well. His current doses are 7 units of Lispro and 22 units of Lantus each morning. Since the diagnosis of metabolic syndrome Rick has been taking Lasix and Lopressor.

History of Current Illness: Rick was taking out the trash and recycling bins one week ago and stepped on a sharp rock. This rock punctured a 1½ cm cut into his right heel. Since this time the foot has become progressively more painful and the small cut has grown to the size of 3 cm in diameter. Rick has had a hard time controlling his blood sugar levels since he cut his foot. Prior to this event Rick's blood glucose levels were consistently in the 140–160 mg/dL range. Since receiving the cut Rick has not been able to get his blood glucose levels below 180 mg/dL. His doctor tried offering Rick additional insulin to assist with blood sugar control, however, this additional insulin did not appear to help lower overall blood sugar levels. Rick saw his doctor three days after cutting his foot and oral clindamycin was started. At today's follow-up appointment, one week after the cut, Rick's doctor noticed necrotic areas surrounding the entire wound. Ricks toes appeared to have a grey tint to them. Rick's foot appeared colder than normal. Due to the progression and current status of the wound, Rick's doctor wanted to admit him to the hospital for IV antibiotics and surgical debridement. Rick was told to go home, pack a bag and report directly to the local hospital.

Anthropometrics in the Doctor's Office:

Height: 6 feet tall; current weight: 239lbs. Weight at last doctor's appointment two weeks ago: 245lbs.

Waist measurement: 44 inches

Body composition information and nutrition focused physical exam: Data unavailable

Hand grip strength with dynamometer: Normal limits for age

Typical Dietary Intake Reported at Doctor's Office: Overall, Rick has been compliant with his dietary modifications. He occasionally consumes some salty foods but this is Rick's only report of dietary "cheating." Rick reports a poor appetite for the past five days. While Rick does try to consume three meals per day, he reports that his portions have decreased since cutting his foot. He does try to consume some protein with each meal; however, he has preferred the taste of fruited yogurt, cottage cheese, cheese, or scrambled eggs with salt instead of meat since cutting his foot.

Hospital Admit and Day 2: Upon admit the MD ordered a "high protein, low sodium, CHO-controlled" diet. Rick ate 40% of his evening meal. Rick was npo after midnight for surgery the next morning. Rick was taken to the operating room on hospital day 2 for wound debridement. The surgeon removed quite a bit of necrotic tissue and the size of the wound on Rick's heel increased to approximately 4.5 cm in diameter. The edges of the wound appeared questionable post-op and the surgeon told Rick's wife that further debridement is likely. He was concerned for both the tissue surrounding the wound as well as the possibility of osteomyelitis. Rick returned to his room post-op and his diet was advanced. Days 1–2 medications included Metformin, Glipizide, Lantis, Lopressor, Lasix, Percocet, IV metronidazole, and IV vancomycin. He received a ½ NS IV at 70 mL/hr to promote adequate urinary output.

Table 4.6: Fasting Comprehensive Metabolic Panel, BUN/Creatinine and A/G Ratios and Osmolality Obtained on Days 1 and 5. Rick Was Fasting 5 Hours Before Day 1 Labs Were Obtained.

Laboratory Values	Normal Ranges or Values	Rick's Laboratory Values: Admit	Rick's Laboratory Values Day 5	Rick's Trend (Improving, Stable, Worsening)	Implications or Assessment
Glucose, mg/dL	70–110	208	153		
Sodium mEq/L	136–145	142	138		
Potassium, mEq/L	3.5–5.0	4.7	3.8		
Chloride, mEq/L	98–106	103	101		
CO_2, mEq/L	23–30	29	25		
BUN, mg/dL	10–20	24	18		
Creatinine, mg/dL	Male: 0.6–1.2	1.3	0.9		
BUN/Creatinine ratio	10–20	18.5	20		
Calcium, mg/dL	9.0–10.5	9.3	9.5		
Albumin, g/d	3.5–5.0	3.0	3.2		
Total protein, g/dL	6.4–8.3	6.4	6.2		
Globulin, g/dL	2.3–3.4	3.9	3.4		
Albumin/Globulin ratio	>1.0	0.77	0.94		
Bilirubin, total, mg/dL	0.3–1.0	0.8	1.0		
ALP, U/L	30–120	120	124		
ALT, U/L	4–36	31	32		
AST, U/L	0–35	30	32		
Osmolality, mOsm/Kg H_2O	285–295	298	288		

Table 4.7: Selected Values from CBC with Differential Obtained on Days 1 and 5. Rick Was Fasting 5 Hours Before Day 1 Labs Were Obtained.

Laboratory Values	Normal Ranges or Values	Rick's Laboratory Values: Admit	Rick's Laboratory Values Day 5	Rick's Trend (Improving, Stable, Worsening)	Implications or Assessment
Hemoglobin, g/dL	Male: 14–18	15	16		
Hematocrit, %	Male: 42–52	44	44		
WBC, SI units	5–10	14.7	12.0		
Neutrophils, %	55–70	102	95		
Platelet count, SI units	150–400	365	350		

Table 4.8: Lipid Panel Obtained Upon Admit to the Hospital. Rick Was Fasting 5 Hours Before Labs Were Obtained.

Laboratory Values	Normal Ranges or Values	Rick's Values	Rick's Value (WNL, High or Low)	Implications or Assessment
Triglycerides, mg/dL	Male: 40–160	220		
HDL cholesterol, mg/dL	Male: >45	40		
LDL cholesterol, mg/dL	60–180	180		
Total cholesterol, mg/dL	<200	200		

Table 4.9: Selected Additional Labs and Vital Signs Obtained Upon Admit to the Hospital. Rick Was Fasting 5 Hours Before Labs Were Obtained.

Laboratory Values	Normal Ranges or Values	Rick's Values	Rick's Value (WNL, High or Low)	Implications or Assessment
Prealbumin, mg/dL	15–36	12		
Crp, mg/dL	<1.0	18		
HgbA1C, %	<6.0	8.1		
Temperature, °F	96.4–99.1	102.4		
Blood pressure, mmHg	Systolic <130 Diastolic <85	175/110		
Pulse, beats/minute	60–100	80		
Respirations: breaths/minute	14–20	18		
Pulse oximetry, %	≤95	98		

Hospital Day 4: Rick continued to receive wound care, IV antibiotics, analgesics, hypoglycemic, and blood pressure medications. He received a ½ NS IV at 70 mL/hr to promote adequate urinary output. He received a high protein, low sodium, CHO-controlled diet with an overall average po intake of 20%–35% of his meals and afternoon snack. It was becoming difficult to control Rick's blood sugar levels and the physician added a sliding scale insulin regimen to Rick's daily medication schedule. During dressing changes and wound therapies, Rick could see that his foot was not healing and appeared to be looking worse each day. Rick is not happy about being in the hospital, his backward progress, limited mobility, and no access to his business. His son assured Rick that the business was running well and he should concentrate on recovery and rehabilitation. There were no additional changes in medications, IV fluids or urinary output.

Hospital Day 5: The physician informed Rick that the necrotic area on the foot was continuing to spread. His toes became black and the entire foot was cold. Rick's physician told Rick and his wife that the foot needed to be amputated. He recommended a below-knee amputation (BKA) so Rick could eventually be fitted with a prosthetic device for mobility. While Rick was depressed about this outcome, he could tell that the foot continued to look worse each day. A BKA was scheduled for the next morning. Rick was made npo at midnight in preparation for his surgery at 8:00 a.m. Rick was so upset that he refused his lunch and ate 20% of his dinner that evening. He did continue to take po water well throughout the day. There were no changes in medications, IV fluids, or urinary output.

Hospital Day 6: Rick returned from the operating room after a successful R BKA. Rick's surgeon resumed Rick's high protein, CHO controlled, low sodium diet. Post-op a ½ NS IV at 85 mL/hr was ordered. While he was back in his room in time for a late lunch, Rick refused this meal. He was "not hungry" when dinner arrived. The surgeon was concerned when he checked on Rick during his evening rounds. Rick's lack of po, required nutrition for post-op healing and the overall appearance of weight loss in Rick's face and chest were rationale for suggesting a feeding tube to Rick and his wife. Rick's only reply to this was "fine." Nursing placed a nasogastric tube two hours later and a diabetic tube feeding was initiated at a slow rate. The surgeon ordered a nutrition consult for enteral feeding suggestions and goals for the following morning. Day 6 medications include a morphine sulfate via a patient controlled analgesia (PCA) pump, Lantus, SSI, Lopressor, Lasix, IV metronidazole, and IV vancomycin.

Table 4.10: Fasting Comprehensive Metabolic Panel, BUN/Creatinine and A/G Ratios and Osmolality Obtained on Day 7.

Laboratory Values	Normal Ranges or Values	Rick's Laboratory Values	Rick's Value (WNL, High or Low)	Implications or Assessment
Glucose, mg/dL	70–110	145		
Sodium mEq/L	136–145	137		
Potassium, mEq/L	3.5–5.0	3.8		
Chloride, mEq/L	98–106	98		
CO_2, mEq/L	23–30	28		
BUN, mg/dL	10–20	12		
Creatinine, mg/dL	Male: 0.6–1.2	0.9		
BUN/Creatinine ratio	10–20	13.3		
Calcium, mg/dL	9.0–10.5	9.9		
Albumin, g/d	3.5–5.0	3.1		
Total protein, g/dL	6.4–8.3	6.4		
Globulin, g/dL	2.3–3.4	3.1		
Albumin/Globulin ratio	>1.0	1.0		
Bilirubin, total, mg/dL	0.3–1.0	0.9		
ALP, U/L	30–120	129		
ALT, U/L	4–36	31		
AST, U/L	0–35	22		
Osmolality, mOsm/Kg H_2O	285–295	290		

Table 4.11: Selected Fasting Values from CBC with Differential Obtained on Day 7.

Laboratory Values	Normal Ranges or Values	Rick's Laboratory Values: Admit	Rick's Value (WNL, High or Low)	Implications or Assessment
Hemoglobin, g/dL	Male: 14–18	16		
Hematocrit, %	Male: 42–52	45		
WBC, SI units	5–10	10.7		
Neutrophils, %	55–70	85		
Platelet count SI units	150–400	355		

Hospital Days 7–12: A post-op weight of 96.8 kg was obtained on Rick on the wheelchair scale in the early morning of day 7. On his evening rounds, the surgeon approved your enteral nutrition support goals for Rick. Over the next four days, Rick continued to improve. His RLE stump appeared to be healing well and there were no necrotic areas around the incision. Rick's blood glucose levels stabilized and he was advanced back to a slightly higher dose of his home medications. Rick concluded his course of IV antibiotics and was transitioned to oral antibiotics. Rick was weaned off of the morphine PCA pump and was changed to oral Percocet for pain control. During this time, Rick continued to receive full enteral feedings; however, he was slowly starting to take more food with each subsequent meal. On day 12, during his evening rounds, the surgeon informed Rick that he was going to discontinue the nasogastric feeding tube. As long as Rick progressed and his wound continued to look good over the next twenty-four to thirty-six hours, Rick would be discharged on the morning of day 14.

Case Evaluation

Prioritize Problems and Identify Interprofessional Care

1. List in order of importance Rick's medical/nutritional concerns from admit date through hospital day 5.

2. Review the concerns listed in question 1. Which member of the health-care team should address each concern and how should the concern be addressed?

3. List in order of importance Rick's medical/nutritional concerns on hospital day 7.

4. Review the concerns listed in question 3. Which member of the health-care team should address each concern and how should the concern be addressed?

5. List in order of importance Rick's medical/nutritional concerns on hospital day 13.

6. Review the concerns listed in question 5. Which member of the health-care team should address each concern and how should the concern be addressed?

Disease/Injury Process and Laboratory Interpretation

7. Are there any laboratory values or vital signs upon admit to the hospital that would be a concern with regards to Rick's current condition?

8. What was the significance of Rick's HgbA1C upon admit to the hospital?

9. What is the significance of Rick's overall reported blood sugar levels prior to his admit to the hospital? What do you think is contributing to the hyperglycemia?

10. **a.** Rick has developed metabolic syndrome. Please describe the specific criteria used to diagnose Rick with metabolic syndrome.

   b. How can the diagnosis of metabolic syndrome affect Rick's future health risks?

11. Rick has developed additional complications associated with diabetes. Please describe these additional complications and how they are affecting his current situation.

Anthropometric and Nutrition Assessment

12. a. What is your evaluation of Rick's height/weight status at the doctor's office?

    b. Based on Rick's pre-op body weight, calculate Rick's expected post-op body weight after he underwent the BKA? Does this weight differ from the post-op weight obtained on day 7? Explain why.

13. Upon admit, can Rick be diagnosed with malnutrition based on the ASPEN/AND guidelines? Explain.

14. Assume you performed a nutrition focused physical exam on Rick prior to making your tube feeding recommendations. Describe what you would expect to find in this exam.

15. a. Calculate Rick's total energy and protein requirements upon admit to the hospital. Justify your reasoning for method to determine needs.

    b. Will Rick's energy and protein requirements change post-op? If so reassess and explain your justification.

16. What is your general assessment of Rick's typical dietary intake? Prior to hospital admit do you feel he is consuming adequate, excessive, or deficient energy and protein based on his nutritional requirements? Assess both pre- and postinjury po intake.

17. Can you determine if Rick may have a diet deficient or excessive in micronutrients based on his postinjury dietary intake? Explain.

Medications

18. a. Describe the main functions of Rick's diabetic medications (Metformin, Glipizide, Lispro and Lantus).

    b. Describe any possible adverse side effects or drug-nutrient interactions with these medications.

19. Describe the main functions of Lasix and Lopressor. Describe any possible adverse side effects or drug-nutrient interactions with these medications.

20. Describe the main function of clindamycin. Describe any possible adverse side effects or drug–nutrient interactions with this medication.

21. Describe the main functions of IV metronidazole and IV vancomycin. Describe any possible adverse side effects or drug–nutrient interactions with these medications.

22. Will the Percocet or morphine pose any nutritional concerns for Rick? Explain.

Nutrition Intervention and Recommendations

23. Describe appropriate enteral nutrition therapy for a diabetic patient under these circumstances.

24. Make a recommendation for Rick's goal enteral feedings. Provide nutrition therapy recommendations by citing enteral product, goal rate/hr and daily volume to be infused; total kcal, grams protein, ml free water, %RDI, and grams fiber if indicated.

25. a. Describe how you would like to transition Rick off of enteral nutrition support to a full diet once he starts to increase his oral intake. Do these goals differ from what the surgeon ordered?

    b. Ideally, what percentage of his prescribed diet should Rick be consuming before you consider changing to only nocturnal feedings? Will laboratory values or additional data be considered in this decision?

    c. Ideally, describe when you would discontinue the enteral nutrition support and allow Rick to sustain on po alone. Will laboratory values or additional data be considered in this decision?

Monitoring and Evaluation: Patient Followup-up

26. How often should Rick's tolerance and response to his enteral feedings be evaluated? Explain specifically how you would evaluate tolerance to enteral feeds and labs you would suggest obtaining.

27. Please describe a desired nutritional care follow-up schedule after Rick's hospital discharge and specifically what should be addressed at follow-up assessments or appointments.

28. Do you feel Rick will be compliant with his diet upon discharge? Explain.

Academy of Nutrition and Dietetics (AND) Medical Nutrition Therapy (MNT) Guidelines and Documentation for Dietitians

Nutrition Diagnosis Utilizing the PES Statements:
Prior to day 5:

Day 7:

Day 13:

Nutrition Intervention and Goals Utilizing AND Terminology:
Prior to day 5:

Day 7:

Day 13:

Nutrition Monitoring and Evaluation Utilizing AND Terminology:
Prior to day 5:

Day 7:

Day 13:

REFERENCE LIST

American Diabetes Association, http://www.diabetes.org/.
_____. "Standards of Medical Care in Diabetes 2016." *Diabetes Care*, vol. 39, no. 1, 2016, pp. S1–S106, http://dx.doi.org/10.2337/dc16-S001.
Anne, Van Leeuwen, and Bladh Mickey Lynn. *Davis's Comprehensive Handbook of Laboratory and Diagnostic Tests with Nursing Implications*. 6th ed., F. A. Davis, 2015.
Brown, Benjamin J., and Christopher E. Attinger. "The Below-Knee Amputation: To Amputate or Palliate?" *Advances in Wound Care (New Rochelle)*, vol. 2, no. 1, 2013, pp. 30–35.
Charney, Pamela. "The Nutrition Care Process." *Pocket Guide to Nutrition Assessment*, edited by Pamela Charney and Ainsley Malone, 3rd ed., Academy of Nutrition and Dietetics, 2016, pp. 1–14.

Franz, Marian J., and Allison B. Evert. "Medical Nutrition Therapy for Diabetes Mellitus and Hypoglycemia of Nondiabetic Origin." *Krause's Food and the Nutrition Care Process*, edited by Kathleen Mahn and Janice L. Raymond, 14th ed., Elsevier, 2017.

Jenson, Gordon L., et al. Nutrition Screening and Assessment." *ASPEN Adult Nutrition Support Core Curriculum*, edited by Charles M. Mueller, 2nd ed., American Society of Parenteral and Enteral Nutrition, 2012, pp. 155–69.

Malone, Ainsley, and Carol Hamilton. "The Academy of Nutrition and Dietetics/The American Society for Parenteral and Enteral Nutrition Consensus Malnutrition Characteristics: Application in Practice." *Nutrition in Clinical Practice,* vol. 28, 2013, pp. 639–50.

Merck Manual Professional Version, http://www.merckmanuals.com/professional/.

Nelms, Marcia Nahikian. "Diseases of the Endocrine System." *Nutrition Therapy and Pathophysiology*, edited by Marcia Nahikian-Nelms, 3rd ed., Wadsworth, Cengage Learning, 2016.

Nelms, Marcia, and Habash, Diane. "Nutrition Assessment: Foundation of the Nutrition Care Process." *Nutrition Therapy and Pathophysiology*, edited by Marcia Nahikian-Nelms, 3rd ed., Wadsworth, Cengage Learning, 2016.

Newton, L., and Timothy Garvey. "Nutritional and Medical Management of Diabetes Mellitus in Hospitalized Patients". *ASPEN Adult Nutrition Support Core Curriculum*, edited by Charles Mueller, 2nd ed., American Society of Parenteral and Enteral Nutrition, 2012, pp. 580–602.

Pagana, Kathleen Deska, and Timothy James Pagana. *Mosby's Manual of Diagnostic and Laboratory Tests*. Mosby/Elsevier, 2014.

Peterson, Sarah J. "Nutrition Focused Physical Assessment." *Pocket Guide to Nutrition Assessment*, edited by Pamela Charney and Ainsley Malone, 3rd ed., Academy of Nutrition and Dietetics, 2016, pp. 76–102.

Roberts, S. "Food and Nutrition Related History." *Pocket Guide to Nutrition Assessment, edited by* Pamela Charney and Ainsley Malone, 3rd ed., Academy of Nutrition and Dietetics, 2016, pp. 34–49.

Weledgi, Elroy P., and P. Fokam. "Treatment of the diabetic foot—To amputate or not?" *BMC Surgery*, vol. 14, 2014, p. 83.

CHAPTER **5**

Gastrointestinal Concerns

- -

Case Study: Outpatient with Celiac Disease

Case-Specific Learning Objectives

- ✓ Identify pros and cons of specific diagnostic tests for celiac disease.
- ✓ Identify potential nutritional deficiencies that may develop in individuals with celiac disease and determine appropriate supplementation as indicated.
- ✓ List nutritional and nonnutritional sources of gluten.
- ✓ Plan a gluten-free diet and make appropriate substitutions for gluten containing foods in a typical diet.

Our Patient: Sarah H. is a twenty-one-year-old college junior. She is currently working her way through college and will obtain a degree in education. Her goal is to be a first grade teacher. She currently lives in a small house with two additional roommates. All three students are working their way through college and are mindful of unnecessary expenses. The young women take turns cooking evening meals and always shop the sales for food, toiletries, and cleaning supplies. Due to their busy schedules, the three women have a schedule to split up the cooking, cleaning, and laundry responsibilities.

Three months ago, Sarah was hired as a nanny for a family with four-year-old twins. One of her employers is an architect and the other is an artist. Sarah works for this family three days per week from noon to 6:00 p.m. Every day at work, Sarah prepares lunch for the twins and gives them afternoon snacks. Sarah is pleased that she is able to eat with the twins and believes her overall nutritional intake is improving on the days she works. Since the twin's mother is an artist, they have a small art studio and playroom next to their bedroom. It is filled with assorted art supplies including paper, crayons, colored pencils, colored chalk, watercolors, acrylic paints, glue, stickers, clay, Play Doh, beads, and fabrics. There are four worktables in the room; two for art and two for games. One table always has a puzzle ready to be completed on it. Overall, Sarah considers herself to be moderately active in her job and walking around the college campus.

Medical and Surgical History: Sarah had her appendix removed when she was eight years old. The appendix did not rupture and she was discharged from the hospital the day after surgery. She was diagnosed with anemia when she was fourteen years old and has been taking iron sulfate supplements for the past seven years. She does not smoke or take illicit drugs. Sarah denies any food intolerances or allergies.

Home Medications: Iron sulfate.

History of Current Illness: Over the past three months, Sarah has been becoming progressively fatigued. She feels that her busy work and school schedule play a role in this, but was not sure if her anemia was getting worse. Over the last three months, Sarah reports a variable appetite and has noticed a 10 pound unintentional weight loss. For the past four to five years, Sarah has complained of generalized gastrointestinal (GI) issues. Sometimes, she has problems with constipation or gas. Typically after a bought of constipation, she gets a slight rash on her abdomen and legs. Sarah has always considered herself to have "dry, itchy and sensitive skin" and always uses body lotions to alleviate the dryness. She noticed that her dermatological issues have become worse since she has been in college. Sarah and her roommates only buy lotions, make-up, or laundry detergents that are on sale. She feels that these inexpensive products are making her skin issues worse. She felt she needed to discuss these issues with her family doctor and scheduled an office appointment. The doctor ordered some lab work to be obtained prior to her appointment.

Anthropometrics and Additional Data from Office Exam

Height: 5 feet 6 inches; current weight: 119 pounds; weight three months ago: 129 pounds

Handgrip strength: Average for age

Chest and lungs: Clear, normal breath sounds via auscultation

Heart: Normal rate and rhythm

Eyes and mucous membranes appear moist

Skin and nails: Pallor with koilonychias

Temperature: 98.4°F

Blood pressure: 110/70 mm/Hg

Pulse: 75 beats/min

Respiratory rate: 16 breaths/min

Pulse oximetry: 99%

Table 5.1: Fasting BMP and Osmolality Obtained One Week Prior to Sarah's Doctor Appointment.

Laboratory Value	Normal Ranges or Values	Sarah's Values	Sarah's Value (WNL, High or Low)	Implications or Assessment
Glucose, mg/dL	70–110	95		
BUN, mg/dL	10–20	18		
Creatinine, mg/dL	Female: 0.5–1.1	1.0		
Sodium, mEq/L	136–145	142		
Chloride, mEq/L	98–106	101		
Potassium, mEq/L	3.5–5.0	4.7		
CO2, mEq/L	23–30	27		
Osmolality, mOsm/kg H2O	285–295	289		

Table 5.2: Fasting Selected Values from Complete Blood Count (CBC), Albumin, and Additional Labs Obtained One Week Prior to Sarah's Doctor Appointment.

Laboratory Value	Normal Ranges or Values	Sarah's Values	Sarah's Value (WNL, High or Low)	Implications or Assessment
Hemoglobin, g/dL	Female: 12–16	10		
Hematocrit, %	Female: 37–47	32		
WBC, SI units	5–10	10.2		
Total cholesterol, mg/dL	<200	155		
Albumin, g/dL	3.5–5.0	3.1		
Prealbumin, mg/dL	15–36	13		
CRP, mg/dL	<1.0	5		
HgbA1C, %	<6.0	4.8		
Transferrin, mg/dL	Female: 250–380	391		
Ferritin, ng/mL	Female: 10–150	8		
TIBC, mcg/dL	250–460	473		
Folate, mcg/dL	200–200	178		
Vitamin B12, pg/mL	160–950	147		

Typical Dietary Intake

Breakfast consists of: coffee with creamer and sugar; Greek yogurt and granola/cereal or a bagel, small glass of milk or fresh juice; and a piece of fresh fruit.

Lunch at work with the twins: Macaroni and cheese or some sort of sandwich plus milk and a piece of fruit. They always have cookies or ice cream for dessert.

Dinner at home with the roommates: Baked or grilled meat; usually chicken or fish plus potatoes, rice or pasta, and a large mixed veggie salad with assorted dressings. Evening dessert always consists of fresh or frozen fruit. Sarah does have a glass of beer or wine on weekends.

Sarah usually drinks several glasses of water or plain iced tea with lemon each day. She avoids soft drinks.

Case Evaluation

Disease Process and Laboratory Interpretation

Prioritize Problems and Identify Interprofessional Care

1. List in order of importance Sarah's medical/nutritional concerns.

2. Review the concerns listed in question 1. Which member of the healthcare team should address each concern and how should the concern be addressed?

Disease Process and Laboratory Interpretation

3. What is celiac disease?

4. Is celiac disease a condition that individuals are born with, or are there specific risks or triggers that can promote disease? Explain.

5. Describe how celiac disease causes damage to the small intestine?

6. Describe three different non-GI symptoms of celiac disease.

7. Describe three GI symptoms of celiac disease.

8. Anemia is a common concern in individuals with celiac disease. Explain why.

9. Fat malabsorption may be a concern in individuals with celiac disease. Explain why.

10. Lactose intolerance may be a concern in individuals with celiac disease. Explain why.

11. What type of diet must an individual consume for several weeks prior to testing for celiac disease? Explain.

12. Sarah's family practitioner suspects Sarah may have celiac disease. Additional tests should be performed to confirm this diagnosis. Please describe the following tests, their significance in disease diagnosis and their accuracy among specific populations or age groups.

   a. Small bowel biopsy

   b. Antibodies

   Anti-tissue transglutaminase antibody (tTG–IgA and IgG)

   Antiendomysial antibody (EMA–IgA)

   Antigliadin antibody (AgA–IgG and IgA)

    c. Genetic testing

    Human leukocyte antigen (HLA) DQ2/DQ8

    When is genetic testing appropriate for an individual suspected of having celiac disease?

Anthropometric and Nutrition Assessment

13. What is your overall assessment of Sarah's anthropometric and physical assessment data from her office exam?

14. Calculate Sarah's percentage of weight change over the last three months?

15. Can Sarah be diagnosed with malnutrition based on the ASPEN/AND guidelines? Explain.

16. Calculate Sarah's total energy and protein requirements. Justify your reasoning for method to determine needs.

17. Would you encourage Sarah to gain weight at this time? Explain.

18. What is gluten?

19. Cite what grains are not allowed on a gluten-free diet.

20. Cite what grains are allowed on a gluten-free diet.

21. Describe the rules the Food and Drug Administration (FDA) has set for a type of food to be labeled "gluten free."

22. Are there specific guidelines for alcoholic beverages that are labeled "gluten free?"

23. Do guidelines exist for nonfood type items with regards to labeling them "gluten free?"

24a. An individual has chosen to follow a gluten-free diet because they feel it is a "healthier" diet. What advice do you have for this individual?

24b. Is the person in question 24a at risk of developing nutritional deficiencies by following the gluten-free diet when it is not indicated? Explain.

25. Do individuals who must follow a gluten-free diet have concerns with regards to medications; either over-the-counter or prescription? Explain.

26. What are some nonnutritional sources of gluten that Sarah is exposed to?

Medications

27. Sarah has been taking iron sulfate supplements for years. Are there any other supplements you would recommend and why?

28. Describe any potential GI issues that may be related to the iron sulfate and additional supplements recommended above.

Nutrition Intervention and Recommendations

29. Below are selected foods and beverages from Sarah's typical dietary recall. Determine what foods and beverages are acceptable on a gluten-free diet. Please note a substitute food or beverage for all unacceptable foods.

Food	Cite If Acceptable. If Unacceptable Please Record an Acceptable Food or Beverage
Nondairy coffee creamer	
Bran flakes	
Bagel with cream cheese	
Banana	
1% Milk	
Macaroni and cheese	
Peanut butter	
12-Grain bread	
Chocolate ice cream	
Cookies	
Ranch salad dressing	
Tater tots	
Grilled chicken	
Teriyaki sauce	
Steamed buttered broccoli	
Beer	
Wine	

Monitoring and Evaluation: Patient Follow-Up

30. What is Sarah's long-term prognosis once a gluten-free diet has been implemented and followed for several months?

31. Please describe a desired nutritional care follow-up schedule for Sarah and what should be addressed at follow-up appointments.

32. What specific laboratory values would you like to check after Sarah has been compliant with the gluten-free diet? Describe when and why.

Additional Concerns Related to Celiac Disease and the Gluten-Free Diet

33. Sarah is a female. In the future are there additional possible nutritional-related concerns or disease that may affect her as she approaches menopause? Explain.

Academy of Nutrition and Dietetics (AND) Medical Nutrition Therapy (MNT) Guidelines and Documentation for Dietitians

Nutrition Diagnosis Utilizing the PES Statements:

Nutrition Intervention and Goals Utilizing AND Terminology:

Nutrition Monitoring and Evaluation Utilizing AND Terminology:

REFERENCE LIST

Celiac Disease Foundation. http://www.celiac.org/.

Charney, Pamela. "The Nutrition Care Process." *Pocket Guide to Nutrition Assessment*, edited by Pamela Charney, and Ainsley Malone, 3rd ed., Academy of Nutrition and Dietetics, 2016, pp. 1–14.

Cresi, Gail, and Arlene Escero. "Medical Nutrition Therapy for Lower Gastrointestinal Tract Disorders." *Krause's Food and the Nutrition Care Process*, edited by Kathleen Mahn and Janice L. Raymond, 14th ed., Elsevier, 2017, pp. 525–59.

Franz, Davis, et al. "Gastrointestinal Disease." *ASPEN Adult Nutrition Support Core Curriculum*, edited by Charles M. Mueller, 2nd ed., American Society of Parenteral and Enteral Nutrition, 2012, pp. 426–53.

Gajulapalli, Rama Dilip, and Deepak Pattanshetty. "Coronary Artery Disease Prevalence is Higher among Celiac Disease Patients." Journal of the American College of Cardiology, vol. 63, Suppl. 12, 2014, p. A115. doi:10.1016/S0735-1097(14)60115-7.

Kabbani, Toufic A., et al. "Celiac Disease or Non-celiac Gluten Sensitivity? An Approach to Clinical Differential Diagnosis." *American Journal of Gastroenterology,* vol. 109, 2014, pp. 741–47.

Malone, Ainsley, and Cynthia Hamilton. "The Academy of Nutrition and Dietetics/The American Society for Parenteral and Enteral Nutrition Consensus Malnutrition Characteristics: Application in Practice." *Nutrition in Clinical Practice,* vol. 28, 2013, pp. 639–50.

Merck Manual Professional Version. http://www.merckmanuals.com/professional/nutritional- disorders/ nutrition,-c-,-general-considerations/nutrient-drug-interactions.

Nelms, Marcia. "Diseases of the Lower Gastrointestinal Tract." *Nutrition Therapy and Pathophysiology*, edited by Marcia Nahikian-Nelms, 3rd ed., Wadsworth, Cengage Learning, 2016.

Nelms, Marcia, and Diane Habash. "Nutrition Assessment: Foundation of the Nutrition Care Process." *Nutrition Therapy and Pathophysiology*, edited by Marcia Nahikian-Nelms, 3rd ed., Wadsworth, Cengage Learning, 2016.

NIH Medline Plus. https://www.nlm.nih.gov/medlineplus/magazine/issues/spring15/toc.html.

Pagana, Kathleen Deska, and Timothy James Pagana. *Mosby's Manual of Diagnostic and Laboratory Tests.* Mosby/Elsevier, 2014.

Peterson, Sarah J. "Nutrition Focused Physical Assessment." *Pocket Guide to Nutrition Assessment*, edited by Pamela Charney and Ainsley Malone, 3rd ed., Academy of Nutrition and Dietetics, 2016, pp. 76–102.

van Leeuwen, Anne, and Mickey Lynn Bladh. *Davis's Comprehensive Handbook of Laboratory & Diagnostic Tests with Nursing Implications*, 6th ed., F. A. Davis, 2015.

Case Study: Partial/Subtotal Gastrectomy Following a Sleeve Gastrectomy

Case-Specific Learning Objectives

✓ Assess physical data from a nutrition-focused physical exam.

✓ Plan an appropriate diet considering partial/subtotal gastric resection.

✓ Identify potential nutritional consequences following a partial or subtotal gastrectomy.

✓ Understand the effects of complications associated with obesity.

Our Patient: Gail B. is a forty-two-year-old sedentary female. She is married with four children; the oldest is seventeen and the youngest is nine. She works as an intensive care nurse at a local hospital and her husband is the manager of the Respiratory Therapy department at the same facility. Gail works two to three twelve-hour shifts per week. Her children are all involved in sports. When Gail is not working, she is busy attending her children's sporting events or chauffeuring a group of children to an event or a team practice. Gail is very creative and has been trying to finish all of the scrapbooks she started for each child when they were younger. Gail's husband and all four of her children are considered to be of "normal weight."

Medical and Surgical History: Gail's parents were both overweight and had type 2 diabetes. Gail's father passed away from a heart attack at the age of sixty-one and her mother currently is suffering from complications associated with type 2 diabetes; neuropathy and renal insufficiency.

Gail was physically active as a child and did not start to gain weight until after graduating from nursing school. She does not have any food allergies or aversions and typically eats a wide variety of foods, but prefers not to eat much meat. She reports that there are no foods she dislikes. The snacks and food brought to the nurses from patient families have contributed to Gail's increasing weight. Families typically bring in cookies, donuts, pizza, and boxes of candy for the nurses as a "thank you" for taking care of their loved ones. Periodically, the nurses in Gail's ICU will have weight loss challenges and many will follow the current trending diet. Some of the diets the nursing staff have tried over the years include cabbage soup, hcg, Paleolithic, South Beach, military diet, various cleanses, Atkins, alkaline diet, blood type diet, and the lemonade diet. While the nurses have lost some weight on these diets, they soon gained the weight back.

Gail had the typical childhood ear infections, colds, and strep throat. All of her pregnancies were uneventful; she carried her children to term and had uncomplicated caesarian sections due to three of her children being breech. After each pregnancy, Gail was unable to lose all of her pregnancy weight and her baseline weight subsequently became higher after each pregnancy.

Gail was diagnosed with hypertension five years ago when she was thirty-seven years old. At the time of this diagnosis, she weighed 77.9 kg. Gail requested a nurse educator position in her ICU two years ago as it had become more difficult for Gail to lift patients and stand most of the day due to her increasing weight which was 85.6 kg. Gail currently has pains in her back, both knees, and right hip. Her mobility has decreased due to these issues.

Home Medications: Gail has been taking a calcium channel blocker and angiotensin-converting-enzyme (ACE) inhibitor for the past five years. To deal with the pains in her knees, back, and hip, she has taken ibuprofen and glucosamine for the past two years.

History of Current Illness

For the past year, Gail has been speaking with her physician about having bariatric surgery. Gail has been frustrated with the pains she experiences, her hypertension and her inability to lose weight and keep it off. For the past nine months, Gail has been under the care of a local bariatric surgical facility. She has been attending classes and counseling from a variety of practitioners in preparation for her upcoming gastric sleeve procedure.

Two weeks prior to surgery, Gail underwent a pre-op ECG and additional testing to confirm that *Helicobacter pylori* was not present. The registered dietitian nutritionist (RDN) performed a physical assessment on Gail and noted the following:

Height: 5 feet 4 inches; weight: 91.1 kg

Handgrip strength with dynamometer: Below standard for sex and age

2+ pitting edema bilateral lower extremities

Pallor, dry patches of skin, koilonychia, pale conjunctiva, and gums

A slight depression in the temporalis muscle was noted. Prominent fat pads noted in multiple areas of chest, back, and shoulders.

At this appointment, the RDN once again reviewed the diet and recommended diet progression Gail must follow post-op. Gail reported that she understood all of the information and had no additional questions.

Table 5.3: Fasting BMP and Osmolality Obtained Two Weeks Prior to Gail's Surgery.

Laboratory Value	Normal Ranges or Values	Gail's Values	Gail's Value (WNL, High or Low)	Implications or Assessment
Glucose, mg/dL	70–110	88		
BUN, mg/dL	10–20	13		
Creatinine, mg/dL	Female: 0.5–1.1	0.6		
Sodium, mEq/L	136–145	135		
Chloride, mEq/L	98–106	97		
Potassium, mEq/L	3.5–5.0	3.7		
CO_2, mEq/L	23–30	23		
Osmolality, mOsm/kg H2O	285–295	280		

Table 5.4: Fasting Lipid Panel Obtained Two Weeks Prior to Gail's Surgery.

Laboratory Value	Normal Ranges or Values	Gail's Values	Gail's Value (WNL, High or Low)	Implications or Assessment
Triglycerides, mg/dL	Female: 35–135	140		
HDL, mg/dL	Female: >55	42		
LDL, mg/dL	60–180	154		
Total cholesterol, mg/dL	<200	196		

Table 5.5: Selected Fasting Additional Lab Values and Vital Signs Obtained Two Weeks Prior to Gail's Surgery.

Laboratory Value or Vital Sign	Normal Ranges or Values	Gail's Values	Gail's Value (WNL, High or Low)	Implications or Assessment
Hemoglobin, g/dL	Female: 12–16	11		
Hematocrit, %	Female: 37–47	35		
Ferritin, ng/mL	Female: 10–150	8		
TIBC, mcg/mL	250–460	490		
WBC, SI units	5–10	6.2		
Albumin, g/dL	3.5–5.0	3.5		
Prealbumin, mg/dL	15–36	15		
CRP, mg/dL	<1.0	8.1		
HgbA1C, %	<6.0	5.9		
Temperature, °F	96.4–99.1	98.9		
Blood pressure, mmHg	Systolic <120 Diastolic <80	145/90		
Pulse, beats/minute	60–100	95		
Respirations, breaths/minute	14–20	15		
Pulse oximetry, %	≤95	99		

Hospital Course, Days 1–4: Gail arrived at the local hospital at 6:00 a.m. the day she was scheduled for her laparoscopic sleeve gastrectomy. After surgery, the bariatric surgeon spoke with Gail's husband and told him the surgery went well and Gail would be transferred to her room soon. The surgeon expected Gail to have a normal recovery and anticipated a discharge from the hospital within a few of days. Post-op, Gail was able to ambulate with assistance, use the restroom, and take her ordered diet starting on post-op day 2 without complaints. Gail reported a post-op pain level of four to five on a scale of 10. She remained stable with good pain control and was discharged in the evening on day 4.

Hospital Medications: Gail's surgeon ordered Percocet for pain and continued with her home calcium channel blocker and ACE inhibitor. Gail was discharged on these medications on hospital day 4.

— —

Case Evaluation

Prioritize Problems and Identify Interprofessional Care

1. List in order of importance Gail's medical/nutritional concerns.

2. Review the concerns listed in question 1. Which member of the healthcare team should address each concern and how should the concern be addressed?

Disease Process and Laboratory Interpretation

3. Describe three chronic medical complications associated with obesity?

4. **a.** Gail has developed or is close to developing complications associated with obesity. Name the complications that are currently present.

   b. What complications do you feel Gail could develop in the future, if she does not lose weight? What data are present that show Gail could be at risk for these conditions?

5. Are there laboratory values or vital signs above that would be a concern regarding Gail's condition prior to her gastric sleeve procedure?

6. From a nutritional standpoint, do you agree with Gail receiving a gastric sleeve to promote weight loss? Explain.

7. a. Gail had a sleeve gastrectomy; essentially, she had a partial/subtotal gastrectomy. Describe two other medical conditions that would require someone undergoing a partial/subtotal gastrectomy.

b. Will individuals undergoing a partial/subtotal gastrectomy for the conditions in question 7a also need to be concerned about the diet they follow post-op and in the future? Explain.

Anthropometric and Nutrition Assessment

8. What is your evaluation of Gail's height/weight status prior to the gastric sleeve procedure?

9. What is Gail's percentage of weight change over the last two years?

10. a. Gail reports that she failed weight loss diets in the past because she does not like to eat a lot of meat. What diets did she try that encourage a high meat intake? Explain.

b. Do you feel this is the main reason that Gail failed these diets?

11. a. Describe fad diets and provide two examples of popular fad diets.

    b. What are two flaws associated with fad diets that may limit their success.

    c. Promote your bestselling "latest and greatest" fad diet. What are the characteristics of your diet and how will this diet promote weight loss?

12. a. Can Gail be diagnosed with malnutrition based on the ASPEN/AND guidelines? Explain.

    b. Is it possible for an obese individual to develop malnutrition? Explain.

13. a. Calculate Gail's total energy and protein requirements after her surgical procedure. Justify your reasoning for method to determine needs.

    b. Could there be several different caloric and protein goals for Gail based on her stage of recovery or time post sleeve gastrectomy. Explain.

    c. Do you feel it will be a challenge for Gail to meet her energy and protein requirements to promote healing after her surgery? Explain.

Medications

14. Describe the main functions of calcium channel blockers and ACE inhibitors. Describe any possible adverse side effects or drug–nutrient interactions with these medications.

15. Describe the main function of glucosamine. Describe possible adverse side effects or drug–nutrient interactions with this medication.

16. Describe the main functions of ibuprofen and Percocet. Describe possible adverse side effects or drug–nutrient interactions with these medications.

Nutrition Intervention and Recommendations

17. Describe the unique properties of each stage of the diet Gail must follow after her sleeve gastrectomy.

a. Immediately post-op

b. Next stage approximately four days after her initial post-op diet

c. Next stage approximately two to three weeks post-op

d. Final advancement at approximately four plus weeks post-op

18. Regardless of the reason for the partial or subtotal gastrectomy, what are some complications associated with noncompliance to dietary modifications following a partial or subtotal gastrectomy?

19. Gail will need to comply with dietary modifications following her surgery. Please develop a sample meal plan for Gail as she recovers and resumes her new eating patterns. Make sure the meal plan is balanced, an appropriate consistency for Gail's postoperative status, allows for adequate fluids and snacks at appropriate times. Make sure all approximate portion sizes are included as well.

Food/Meal	Recommended Diet for Gail 1–3 Days Post-op	Recommended Diet for Gail 4–14 Days Post-op (Approx. Duration)	Recommended Diet for Gail 2–3 Weeks Post-op (Approx. Duration)	Recommended Diet for Gail 4+ Weeks Post-op (Approx. Duration)
Breakfast				
Midmorning snack				
Lunch				
Midafternoon snack				
Dinner				
Evening snack				

20. a. Gail is at risk for developing nutritional deficiencies after her sleeve gastrectomy. What nutrient deficiencies may develop in the future?

b. Describe possible chronic conditions that may develop in Gail after this procedure?

c. Describe the specific micronutrient supplementation you would recommend to minimize nutritional risks in Gail?

Monitoring and Evaluation: Patient Follow-Up

21. Please describe a desired nutritional care follow-up schedule for Gail. What should be addressed at follow-up appointments.

22. What specific questions would you ask Gail at her follow-up appointments to see if she understands the prescribed diet advancement?

23. Do you feel Gail will be compliant with her diet upon discharge? Explain.

Academy of Nutrition and Dietetics (AND) Medical Nutrition Therapy (MNT) Guidelines and Documentation for Dietitians

Nutrition Diagnosis Utilizing the PES Statements:

Nutrition Intervention and Goals Utilizing AND Terminology:

Nutrition Monitoring and Evaluation Utilizing AND Terminology:

REFERENCE LIST

Academy of Nutrition and Dietetics. http://www.eatright.org/resources/health/weight-loss/fad-diets.

American Heart Association. http://www.heart.org/.

American Society for Bariatric and Metabolic Surgery. https://asmbs.org/.

Charney, Pamela. "The Nutrition Care Process." *Pocket Guide to Nutrition Assessment*, edited by Pamela Charney, and Ainsley Malone, 3rd ed., Academy of Nutrition and Dietetics, 2016, pp. 1–14.

Cresi, Gail, and Arlene Escero. "Medical Nutrition Therapy for Lower Gastrointestinal Tract Disorders." *Krause's Food and the Nutrition Care Process*, edited by Kathleen Mahn and Janice L. Raymond, 14th ed., Elsevier, 2017, pp. 525–59.

Geraci, Angela, et al. "The Work behind Weight-Loss Surgery: A Qualitative Analysis of Food Intake after the First Two Years Post-Op." *ISRN Obesity*, vol. 2014, 2014, p. 427062. doi:10.1155/2014/427062.

Hart, Ryan T., and Thomas H. Frazier. "Obesity." *ASPEN Adult Nutrition Support Core Curriculum*, edited by Charles M. Mueller, 2nd ed., American Society of Parenteral and Enteral Nutrition, 2012, pp. 603–19.

Malone, Ainsley, and Cynthia Hamilton. "The Academy of Nutrition and Dietetics/The American Society for Parenteral and Enteral Nutrition Consensus Malnutrition Characteristics: Application in Practice." *Nutrition in Clinical Practice*, vol. 28, 2013, pp. 639–50.

Merck Manual Professional Version. http://www.merckmanuals.com/professional.

Nelms, Marcia. "Diseases of the Lower Gastrointestinal Tract." *Nutrition Therapy and Pathophysiology*, edited by Marcia Nahikian-Nelms, 3rd ed., Wadsworth, Cengage Learning, 2016.

Nelms, Marcia, and Diane Habash. "Nutrition Assessment: Foundation of the Nutrition Care Process." *Nutrition Therapy and Pathophysiology*, edited by Marcia Nahikian-Nelms, 3rd ed., Wadsworth, Cengage Learning, 2016.

NIH National Library of Medicine Drug Information. https://www.nlm.nih.gov/medlineplus/druginfo/.

Pagana, Kathleen Deska, and Timothy James Pagana. *Mosby's Manual of Diagnostic and Laboratory Tests*. Mosby/Elsevier, 2014.

Peterson, Sarah J. "Nutrition Focused Physical Assessment." *Pocket Guide to Nutrition Assessment*, edited by Pamela Charney and Ainsley Malone, 3rd ed., Academy of Nutrition and Dietetics, 2016, pp. 76–102.

Roberts, Susan. "Food and Nutrition Related History." *Pocket Guide to Nutrition Assessment,* edited by Pamela Charney and Ainsley Malone, 3rd ed., Academy of Nutrition and Dietetics, 2016, pp. 34–49.

van Leeuwen, Anne, and Mickey Lynn Bladh. *Davis's Comprehensive Handbook of Laboratory & Diagnostic Tests with Nursing Implications*, 6th ed., F. A. Davis, 2015.

Case Study: Diverticular Disease

Case-Specific Learning Objectives

✓ Plan an appropriate diet considering exacerbation and remission of diverticular disease.

✓ Evaluate ethnic variations of dietary modifications

Our Patient: Steve P. is a fifty-four-year-old male of South American decent. His parents immigrated to the United States shortly after they married. He is divorced, has one grown daughter who became engaged two months ago and is planning a big wedding in five months. Recently, Steve feels that he has been acting as a referee between his daughter and ex-wife regarding wedding plans as they have had trouble agreeing on most decisions.

Steve has been employed at the same company since graduating college in his early 20's as an electrical engineer and has advanced to middle management. Steve's company announced an upcoming reorganization one month before his daughter announced her engagement. Steve typically works out at the gym four to five days per week before going to work. Over the past three weeks, Steve has missed many of his morning workouts due to arriving earlier than usual at work.

Steve loves to work in his yard and garden and has been taking care of his mother's yard since his dad passed away three years ago. Steve enjoys cooking and preparing what he harvests from his garden. Steve is not a heavy drinker, but will have mixed drinks if out with or entertaining friends on weekends. For the past two weeks, Steve has had a bottle of beer each night after arriving home from work. He will drink soda or iced tea during the day; he has never been a big water drinker as he prefers beverages with flavor.

Medical and Surgical History: Steve had the typical childhood illnesses. He was very active as a child and received a couple of cuts that required stitches. He did not break any bones, but did sprain his ankle twice playing basketball.

Steve's father passed away from complications associated with type 2 diabetes. His mother is healthy, active, and has no major health concerns except for osteoporosis. Steve has one brother and one sister and both are healthy, active, and normal weight. Steve's brother has had annual colonoscopies and a benign polyp removal four years ago and his sister has osteopenia. Steve was diagnosed with diverticulosis four years ago when he underwent his first screening colonoscopy. His doctor advised Steve to exercise, drink plenty of water, and see a dietitian for nutrition education regarding what to eat now and in the future if the diverticula become irritated or infected.

Home Medications: None.

History of Current Illness: Steve noticed dull diffuse abdominal pain six days ago. Over the next couple of days, the pain became progressively worse; especially after meals. Two days ago, Steve noticed he was becoming constipated and felt chills. Steve wanted to eat, but his appetite was poor. This morning when Steve woke up he felt nauseated, his abdominal pain was worse, he was constipated, and had a fever of 102.5°F. He ate a small bowl of oatmeal and had some apple juice before calling his doctor for an appointment. Steve was able to get an appointment to see his doctor midmorning.

Doctor's Office Visit: Steve was uncomfortable when he arrived at his appointment. He reported an abdominal pain level of 5–6 on a scale of 1–10. Steve's abdomen was tender to palpations. The doctor could hear frequent bowel sounds on auscultation. The doctor informed Steve that he was experiencing an episode of diverticulitis and wanted to get a CT scan of the abdomen for confirmation. His doctor ordered a STAT CT scan and blood work. Before Steve left the doctor's office, his blood was drawn. The doctor told Steve that he would call with the CT scan and blood results before his office closed for the day.

At 4:30 p.m., Steve received a call from his doctor's nurse informing him that the CT scan confirmed that Steve was experiencing an episode of diverticulitis. Prescriptions for ciprofloxacin, metronidazole, and tylenol with codeine were called into the local pharmacy. Steve was advised to follow his liquid, low residue diet recommendations and follow-up with the doctor in a week.

Typical Dietary Intake: Steve reports he eats meat or a "decent source of protein" at every meal.

Breakfast: He likes omelets in the mornings and mixes in a variety of meats, cheeses, and vegetables. Otherwise, he will eat a bagel with nut butter, scrambled eggs, and fruit. Steve has a couple cups of black coffee each morning.

Lunch: Steve eats a large meat sandwich (chicken, turkey, or roast beef with cheese, veggies, and mayonnaise) or any kind of fast food on weekdays. He always packs a couple of servings of fruit to take to the office to eat each day. Steve likes iced tea for lunch. Recently on weekends, Steve has been so busy or preoccupied that he may skip lunch. He will snack on whatever he finds in his pantry or fridge all day. Steve admits to eating more cookies,. pastries and ice cream recently.

Dinner: Steve likes to try new sauces and marinades, so he will use these on baked or grilled meat; usually chicken, pork chops, steak, or fish. Steve will have a large slice of whole grain bread and potatoes, rice or pasta, plus a mixed veggie salad with assorted dressings or steamed vegetables. Steve reports that he has been craving the foods he ate as a child and has been consuming more fish, chicken, rice, and beans using his mother's recipes. Recently, Steve has been having a bottle of beer with dinner and he will always have a glass of water. Steve will eat a small dessert each evening, usually favoring cookies.

Anthropometrics and Additional Data from Office Exam

Height: 5 feet 9 inches; current weight: 197 pounds

Handgrip strength: Average for age

Chest and lungs: Clear, normal breath sounds via auscultation

Heart: Normal rate and rhythm

Eyes and mucous membranes appear moist

Temperature, °F: 103.3

Blood pressure, mmHg: 140/80

Pulse, beats/minute: 90

Respirations, breaths/minute: 16

Pulse oximetry: 98%

Table 5.6: Nonfasting Comprehensive Metabolic Panel, Albumin/Globulin (A/G) Ratio, CRP, HgbA1C, and Osmolality Obtained at Doctor's Office.

Laboratory Value	Normal Ranges or Values	Steve's Laboratory Values	Steve's Value (WNL, High or Low)	Implications or Assessment
Glucose, mg/dL	70–110	148		
Sodium, mEq/L	136–145	142		
Potassium, mEq/L	3.5–5.0	4.8		
Chloride, mEq/L	98–106	103		
CO_2, mEq/L	23–30	27		
BUN, mg/dL	10–20	15		
Creatinine, mg/dL	Male: 0.6–1.2	0.9		
Calcium, mg/dL	9.0–10.5	9.4		
Albumin, g/dL	3.5–5.0	3.7		
Total protein, g/dL	6.4–8.3	7.9		
Globulin, g/dL	2.3–3.4	3.3		
A/G ratio	>1.0	1.03		
Bilirubin, total, mg/dL	0.3–1.0	0.8		
ALP, U/L	30–120	110		
ALT, U/L	4–36	25		
AST, U/L	0–35	28		
Osmolality, mOsm/kg H_2O	285–295	292		
CRP, mg/dL	<1.0	15		
HgbA1C	<6.0	4.9		

Table 5.7: Selected Nonfasting Values from CBC and Differential Obtained at Doctor's Office.

Laboratory Values	Normal Ranges or Values	Steve's Laboratory Values	Steve's Value (WNL, High or Low)	Implications or Assessment
Hemoglobin, g/dL	Male: 14–18	16		
Hematocrit, %	Male: 42–52	44		
WBC, SI units	5–10	12.2		
Lymphocytes, %	20–40	44		
Neutrophils, %	55–70	82		
Platelet count SI units	150–400	255		

Case Evaluation

Prioritize Problems and Identify interprofessional Care

1. List in order of importance Steve's medical/nutritional concerns.

2. Review the concerns listed in question 1 above. Which member of the health-care team should address each concern and how should the concern be addressed?

Disease Process, Laboratory Interpretation, and Diagnosis

3. What is diverticulosis?

4. What is diverticulitis?

5. Describe complications associated with diverticular disease.

6. How is diverticular disease diagnosed?

7. What are the signs and symptoms of diverticulitis? Are any of these present in Steve's case?

8. a. Are there specific risk factors for developing diverticular disease? Explain.

b. Are any of these risk factors present in Steve? Explain.

9. Are there laboratory values or vital signs above that would be a concern regarding to Steve's condition? Explain.

10. In cases of complications arising from diverticulitis, a partial bowel resection may need to be performed to remove the damaged and infected bowel. In some cases, a colostomy or ileostomy will be performed in conjunction with this partial colon resection.
a. What is a colostomy?

b. Describe the nutritional and diet concerns of someone who has a colostomy.

c. What is an ileostomy?

    d. Describe the nutritional and diet concerns of someone who has an ileostomy.

    e. Describe why an individual with an ileostomy is at risk for developing dehydration and electrolyte imbalances.

Anthropometric and Nutrition Assessment

11. What is your evaluation of Steve's current height/weight status?

12. Can Steve be diagnosed with malnutrition based on the ASPEN/AND guidelines? Explain.

13. a. Calculate Steve total energy and protein requirements? Justify your reasoning for method to determine needs.

    b. Will these energy and protein requirements change once the diverticulitis is in remission? Explain

14. What is your general assessment of Steve's typical dietary intake? Do you feel that he is consuming adequate, excessive or deficient energy and protein based on his nutritional requirements?

15. Can you determine if Steve may have a diet deficient in micronutrients based on his current typical dietary intake? Explain.

16. What is your evaluation of the fiber and fluid content of Steve's typical diet based on his typical dietary intake?

Medications

17. Describe the main function of ciprofloxacin and metronidazole. Describe possible adverse side effects or drug–nutrient interactions with these medications.

18. Describe the main function of Tylenol with codeine. Describe possible adverse side effects or drug–nutrient interactions with this medication.

Nutrition Intervention and Recommendations

19. Describe the appropriate diet therapy for diverticulitis.

20. Describe the appropriate diet therapy for diverticulosis that Steve will need to follow once the diverticulitis is resolved.

21. Based on Steve's typical dietary intake, please develop a diet for Steve to follow for his diverticulosis and whenever he has a flare-up of his condition.

Food/Meal	Recommended Diet for Diverticulitis	Recommended Diet for Diverticulosis
Breakfast		
Lunch		
Dinner		

Food/Meal	Recommended Diet for Diverticulitis	Recommended Diet for Diverticulosis
Optional snacks		

Monitoring and Evaluation: Patient Follow-Up

22. Please describe a desired nutritional care follow-up schedule for Steve and what should be addressed at follow-up appointments.

23. What specific questions will you ask Steve in a follow-up to see if he understands his prescribed diet?

Academy of Nutrition and Dietetics (AND) Medical Nutrition Therapy (MNT) Guidelines and Documentation for Dietitians

Nutrition Diagnosis Utilizing the PES Statements:

Nutrition Intervention and Goals Utilizing AND Terminology:

Nutrition Monitoring and Evaluation Utilizing AND Terminology:

REFERENCE LIST

Charney, Pamela. "The Nutrition Care Process." *Pocket Guide to Nutrition Assessment*, edited by Pamela Charney, and Ainsley Malone, 3rd ed., Academy of Nutrition and Dietetics, 2016, pp. 1–14.

Cresi, Gail, and Arlene Escero. "Medical Nutrition Therapy for Lower Gastrointestinal Tract Disorders." *Krause's Food and the Nutrition Care Process*, edited by Kathleen Mahn and Janice L. Raymond, 14th ed., Elsevier, 2017, pp. 525–59.

Malone, Ainsley, and Cynthia Hamilton. "The Academy of Nutrition and Dietetics/The American Society for Parenteral and Enteral Nutrition Consensus Malnutrition Characteristics: Application in Practice." *Nutrition in Clinical Practice*, vol. 28, 2013, pp. 639–50.

Merck Manual Professional Version. http://www.merckmanuals.com/professional.

Nelms, Marcia. "Diseases of the Lower Gastrointestinal Tract." *Nutrition Therapy and Pathophysiology*, edited by Marcia Nahikian-Nelms, 3rd ed., Wadsworth, Cengage Learning, 2016.

Nelms, Marcia, and Diane Habash. "Nutrition Assessment: Foundation of the Nutrition Care Process." *Nutrition Therapy and Pathophysiology*, edited by Marcia Nahikian-Nelms, 3rd ed., Wadsworth, Cengage Learning, 2016.

NIH National Library of Medicine Drug Information. https://www.nlm.nih.gov/medlineplus/druginfo/.

Pagana, Kathleen Deska, and Timothy James Pagana. *Mosby's Manual of Diagnostic and Laboratory Tests*. Mosby/Elsevier, 2014.

Roberts, Susan. "Food and Nutrition Related History." *Pocket Guide to Nutrition Assessment*, edited by Pamela Charney and Ainsley Malone, 3rd ed., Academy of Nutrition and Dietetics, 2016, pp. 34–49.

van Leeuwen, Anne, and Mickey Lynn Bladh. *Davis's Comprehensive Handbook of Laboratory & Diagnostic Tests with Nursing Implications*, 6th ed., F. A. Davis, 2015.

Case Study: Hiatal Hernia and GERD (Gastroesophageal Reflux Disease)

Case-Specific Learning Objectives

- ✓ Plan an appropriate diet considering the presence of a hiatal hernia and gastroesophageal reflux disease (GERD).
- ✓ Recommend appropriate lifestyle modifications considering the presence of a hiatal hernia and GERD.
- ✓ Evaluate ethnic variations of dietary modifications

Our Patient: Carol V. is a forty-three-year-old female of Italian decent. Her family immigrated to the United States shortly after Carol's fifteenth birthday. She is married and has one college age son.

Carol has been employed as a junior high school science teacher since graduating from college in her early 20s. Carol does not like "moving fast and sweating." She started taking yoga classes six months ago and feels this has helped her overall well being and ability to relax. Carol enjoys cooking and baking. She will drink water or iced tea during the day, but prefers diet cola. She does smoke one pack of cigarettes every two to three days.

Medical and Surgical History: Carol had the typical childhood illnesses. She was very active as a child but had no major injuries. Carol's pregnancy and delivery were uneventful. Carol's mother passed away from complications associated with cardiovascular disease and obesity. Her father is healthy, active, and has no major health concerns. Carol has two sisters; both are healthy and one is obese.

Home Medications: Over-the-counter acid reducers. Carol has tried a variety of these products and none seem to help (for example, Tums, Pepcid, Prilosec).

History of Current Illness: Over the past four months, Carol noticed abdominal pain and "heartburn" after eating; especially after her evening meal. The pain started as dull and has become progressively worse. Carol likes most foods and it appears that eating in general causes heartburn. The pain seems to get worse right after eating. Carol's appetite has decreased over the past three weeks due to overall pain with eating. Carol reports that she has not weighed herself, but feels like she has lost weight. Her clothes appear to have become a little looser on her body. Carol has not had any issues with emesis, diarrhea, or constipation. Due to recurrent issues of heartburn and no relief from over-the-counter remedies, Carol has decided to see her doctor to see if something could be done about her pain after eating. Carol's doctor ordered fasting blood work and referred her to a gastroenterologist for an upper GI endoscopy to determine the cause of her persistent heartburn.

Table 5.8: Fasting BMP, Osmolality, Albumin, and Hgb A1C Obtained at Doctor's Office.

Laboratory Value	Normal Ranges or Values	Carol's Values	Carol's Value (WNL, High or Low)	Implications or Assessment
Glucose, mg/dL	70–110	75		
BUN, mg/dL	10–20	15		
Creatinine, mg/dL	Feale: 0.5–1.1	0.9		
Sodium, mEq/L	136–145	140		
Chloride, mEq/L	98–106	100		
Potassium, mEq/L	3.5–5.0	4.8		
CO_2, mEq/L	23–30	27		
Osmolality, mOsm/kg H_2O	285–295	284		
Albumin, g/dL	3.5–5.0	3.7		
CRP, mg/dL	<1.0	0.4		

Table 5.9: Selected Fasting Values from Complete Blood Count and Differential Obtained at Doctor's Office.

Laboratory Values	Normal Ranges or Values	Carol's Laboratory Values:	Carol's Value (WNL, High or Low)	Implications or Assessment
Hemoglobin, g/dL	Female: 12–16	13		
Hematocrit, %	Female: 37–47	40		
WBC, SI units	5–10	8.4		
Lymphocytes, %	20–40	33		
Neutrophils, %	55–70	59		
Platelet count SI units	150–400	268		

Appointment with Gastroenterologist: Three weeks later, Carol underwent an upper gastrointestinal (UGI) endoscopy and had a chest x-ray taken. She had a follow-up appointment with the gastroenterologist a week later where test results were discussed. The gastroenterologist reported Carol's stomach lining appeared normal. A hiatal hernia was present and there was some irritation of the lower esophageal tissue close to the hiatal hernia. He prescribed omeprazole and referred Carol to a dietitian for nutritional advice.

Typical Dietary Intake

Breakfast: Carol likes coffee, pastries, and fruits in the mornings. Occasionally, she will have some meat or cheese with bread. Carol does not like cereal or milk.

Lunch: Carol likes to have some sort of soup or meat, cheese, and crackers for lunch. She will occasionally have a big hot meal. She also likes salads with a variety of raw veggies, meat, cheese, and hard boiled eggs. Carol prefers a balsamic vinaigrette salad dressing.

Dinner: Carol cooks a big Italian meal for dinner and serves large portions. She likes pastas, meats, seafood, vegetables and always adds a lot of fresh garlic, basil, and oregano to her meals. Carol will eat a small dessert each evening before bed, usually favoring cake and gelato. Carol does not eat much fruit. Due to Carol's family traditions, she is accustomed to having a glass of red wine with dinner each evening.

Anthropometrics and Additional Data from Gastroenterologist's Exam

Height: 5 feet 5 inches; current weight: 167 pounds

Handgrip strength: Average for age

Chest and lungs: Clear, normal breath sounds via auscultation

Heart: Normal rate and rhythm

Eyes and mucous membranes appear moist

Temperature, °F: 98.3

Blood pressure, mmHg: 130/70

Pulse, beats/minute: 90

Respirations, breaths/minute: 16

Pulse oximetry: 100%

Case Evaluation

Prioritize Problems and Identify interprofessional Care

1. List in order of importance Carol's medical/nutritional concerns.

2. Review the concerns listed in question 1 above. Which member of the health-care team should address each concern and how should the concern be addressed?

Disease Process and Laboratory Interpretation

3. What is a hiatal hernia?

4. What is GERD?

5. Describe complications associated with a hiatal hernia and GERD?

6. a. What are the signs and symptoms of a hiatal hernia and GERD ? Are any of these present in Carol's case?

b. Are there specific risk factors for developing a hiatal hernia and GERD? Explain

c. Are any of these risk factors present in Carol? Explain.

7. Are there laboratory values or vital signs above that would be a concern regarding Carol's condition? Explain.

Anthropometric and Nutrition Assessment

8. What is your evaluation of Carol's current height/weight status?

9. Can Carol be diagnosed with malnutrition based on the ASPEN/AND guidelines? Explain.

10. Calculate Carol's total energy and protein requirements? Justify your reasoning for method to determine needs.

11. What is your general assessment of Carol's typical dietary intake? Do you feel that she is consuming adequate, excessive or deficient energy and protein based on her nutritional requirements?

12. Can you determine if Carol may have a diet deficient in micronutrients based on her typical dietary intake? Explain.

13. Can you determine if Carol may be consuming foods or beverages that may contribute to the adverse symptoms associated with a hiatal hernia and GERD? Explain.

Medications

14. Describe the main functions of over-the-counter acid reducing agents. Describe possible adverse side effects or drug–nutrient interactions with these medications.

Nutrition Intervention and Recommendations

15. Describe the appropriate diet therapy for a hiatal hernia. Explain.

16. Based on Carol's typical dietary intake, please develop a diet for Carol to follow to alleviate the adverse symptoms associated with a hiatal hernia. Note if an item Carol typically consumes is acceptable or not for her condition.

Food/Beverage and Recommended Time of Consumption	Acceptable to Consume with Carol's Current Condition? Yes or No	Substitution to Help Alleviate Carol's Adverse Symptoms (If Applicable)
Breakfast		
Lunch		
Dinner		

Food/Beverage and Recommended Time of Consumption	Acceptable to Consume with Carol's Current Condition? Yes or No	Substitution to Help Alleviate Carol's Adverse Symptoms (If Applicable)
Optional snacks		

Monitoring and Evaluation: Patient Follow-Up

17. Please describe a desired nutritional care follow-up schedule for Carol and what should be addressed at follow-up appointments.

18. What specific questions will you ask Carol in a follow-up to see if she understands his prescribed diet?

Academy of Nutrition and Dietetics (AND) Medical Nutrition Therapy (MNT) Guidelines and Documentation for Dietitians

Nutrition Diagnosis Utilizing the PES Statements:

Nutrition Intervention and Goals Utilizing AND Terminology:

Nutrition Monitoring and Evaluation Utilizing AND Terminology:

REFERENCE LIST

Charney, Pamela. "The Nutrition Care Process." *Pocket Guide to Nutrition Assessment*, edited by Pamela Charney, and Ainsley Malone, 3rd ed., Academy of Nutrition and Dietetics, 2016, pp. 1–14.

Cresi, Gail, and Arlene Escero. "Medical Nutrition Therapy for Lower Gastrointestinal Tract Disorders." *Krause's Food and the Nutrition Care Process*, edited by Kathleen Mahn and Janice L. Raymond, 14t7h ed., Elsevier, 2017, pp. 525–59.

Malone, Ainsley, and Cynthia Hamilton. "The Academy of Nutrition and Dietetics/The American Society for Parenteral and Enteral Nutrition Consensus Malnutrition Characteristics: Application in Practice." *Nutrition in Clinical Practice,* vol. 28, 2013, pp. 639–50.

Merck Manual Professional Version. http://www.merckmanuals.com/professional.

Nelms, Marcia. "Diseases of the Lower Gastrointestinal Tract." *Nutrition Therapy and Pathophysiology*, edited by Marcia Nahikian-Nelms, 3rd ed., Wadsworth, Cengage Learning, 2016.

Nelms, Marcia, and Diane Habash. "Nutrition Assessment: Foundation of the Nutrition Care Process." *Nutrition Therapy and Pathophysiology*, edited by Marcia Nahikian-Nelms, 3rd ed., Wadsworth, Cengage Learning, 2016.

NIH National Library of Medicine Drug Information. https://www.nlm.nih.gov/medlineplus/druginfo/.

Pagana, Kathleen Deska, and Timothy James Pagana. *Mosby's Manual of Diagnostic and Laboratory Tests*. Mosby/Elsevier, 2014.

Roberts, Susan. "Food and Nutrition Related History." *Pocket Guide to Nutrition Assessment,* edited by Pamela Charney and Ainsley Malone, 3rd ed., Academy of Nutrition and Dietetics, 2016, pp. 34–49.

van Leeuwen, Anne, and Mickey Lynn Bladh. *Davis's Comprehensive Handbook of Laboratory & Diagnostic Tests with Nursing Implications*, 6th ed., F. A. Davis, 2015.

Case Study: Patient with Crohn's Disease Requiring Abdominal Surgery and Nutrition Support Therapy.

Case-Specific Learning Objectives

- ✓ Assess risk of developing nutritional deficiencies from long-term GI issues.
- ✓ Plan appropriate parenteral nutrition therapy.
- ✓ Develop cyclic parenteral nutrition therapy
- ✓ Identify characteristics of and plan feeds for prevention of refeeding syndrome.
- ✓ Plan appropriate nutritional therapy to transition from parenteral to oral intake.
- ✓ Evaluate ethnic variations of dietary modifications

Our Patient: Susan P. is a thirty-eight-year-old married female with two children; a six-year-old boy and ten-year-old girl. She works as a self-employed interior designer. Susan is a troop leader for her daughters girl scout troop and is involved as a snack mom for her son's little league team. Her husband is the store manager of a large local grocery store. They own their own home. The family likes to ride bikes and swim. Susan was born in the United States; however, both of her parents were born in Germany.

Medical and Surgical History: Susan suffered from the normal childhood illnesses; had frequent episodes of strep throat while in elementary school and had her tonsils removed when she was in the fifth grade. Susan was relatively healthy until the age of twenty when she started to experience abdominal pain and diarrhea after eating anything containing milk. At this time, she was told she had lactose intolerance and was advised to stop eating all food and beverages containing milk. Susan's symptoms improved for a short while and then the persistent abdominal pain and diarrhea started to get worse. Susan was diagnosed with Crohn's disease when she was twenty-three years old. Since her diagnosis, Susan has undergone multiple endoscopies and colonoscopies. She has had multiple episodes of disease exacerbation over the years and underwent three partial small or large bowel resections in the past. Susan has had a total of 5 feet of small intestine and 4 feet of colon removed to date. She has an intact ileocecal valve, but is missing her entire duodenum. Her first partial small bowel resection was at twenty-four years of age. Since her diagnosis fifteen years ago, Susan has lost a total of 38 pounds based on her current weight. Two years ago Susan tried acupuncture as an alternative therapy to her physician's treatments. She felt better for six months before her pain and diarrhea returned.

Susan had difficulty gaining adequate weight during both pregnancies. Delivery during both pregnancies was via caesarian section at thirty-four weeks gestation. Both children are now healthy, but were born classified as low birth weight.

Home Medications: Tylenol, Metamucil, MVI, Azathioprine.

History of Current Illness: Susan was seen in her doctor's office six days ago due to a flare-up of her Crohn's disease. He prescribed corticosteroids and ciprofloxacin to compliment her daily Crohn's medications. She felt better for a few days but then symptoms resumed and have become progressively worse. Susan complained of diffuse and increasing abdominal pain, fever, chills, diarrhea, and nausea for the past two days. She reports she has lost more weight in the past week. She started vomiting last night and called her doctor's office in the morning. Since it was the weekend, her doctor recommended she report to the local hospital's ER where he would order a CT scan of her abdomen to compliment her ER work-up.

Diet History: Susan had always been a picky eater as a child and went through many food jags as a child and into her teenage years. Susan has had difficulty eating some of her favorite foods ever since her diagnosis of Crohn's disease. These foods include ice cream, citrus, berries, melons, pastries, German sausages, German potato salad, and fast foods from a burger restaurant. She has gone through episodes of being able to tolerate lactose and not being able to tolerate lactose. She can tolerate cooked vegetables and canned or very soft fruits better than raw vegetables and harder fruits like apples. Starches that contain a higher fiber content appear to produce adverse abdominal symptoms. Susan cannot tolerate high fat or fried foods. Due to the multiple foods that have produced adverse abdominal symptoms, Susan has steadily lost weight since her diagnosis. While she is not fond of the taste, she is able to tolerate a commercial oral supplement and always tried to consume at least two of these each day for the past two years. She switches between commercial brands depending on overall price, sales, or the availability of discount coupons. Over the past 2½ weeks, Susan's appetite has decreased and abdominal discomfort has increased. She had only been able to eat a few bites of soft bland foods (scrambled eggs, applesauce, and mashed potatoes) for the last week and has not been able to keep any food down for approximately eight hours prior to hospital admit.

Emergency Room and Hospital Day 1: On presentation to the ER Susan reported sharp abdominal pains. On a pain scale of 1–10, Susan cites the pain until last night was a 4–6 and currently reports the pain is an 8 or 9. The abdominal CT scan revealed an abscess in the jejunum. An incidental notation was recorded on the radiology report of lower than normal psoas muscle mass at the L3 level. She was admitted to the hospital and plans for surgery early in the afternoon were initiated. Susan stated her height is 5 feet 8 inches and she reported weighing 108 pounds one month ago and 103 pounds six days ago in her doctor's office. Susan weighed 112 pounds in the ER.

At 1:00 p.m., Susan was taken to the OR for an exploratory laparotomy and partial small bowel resection. In surgery, the surgeon found more intestinal damage than anticipated. Three feet of Susan's jejunum were resected. The remaining ends of Susan's small intestine near the resected area appeared normal and were anastomosed. Additional areas of the small and large intestine appeared to have "inflammation." Her abdomen was closed. A central line for parenteral nutrition infusion was placed in the OR. Susan was extubated and admitted to the progressive care unit after surgery. Day 1 IV's and medications include D5NS at 100 mL/hr to maintain adequate urine output, prednisone, IV ciprofloxacin, azathioprine, and morphine PCA. Susan received a blood transfusion and 25 grams of 5% IV albumin prior to surgery as well. Susan was npo post-op and the surgeon ordered a nutrition consult for parenteral feeding recommendations.

Table 5.10: Fasting Comprehensive Metabolic Panel, A/G Ratio, and Osmolality Obtained in the ER.

Laboratory Value	Normal Ranges or Values	Susan's Laboratory Values: ER	Susan's Value (WNL, High or Low)	Implications or Assessment
Glucose, mg/dL	70–110	173		
Sodium, mEq/L	136–145	144		
Potassium, mEq/L	3.5–5.0	3.4		
Chloride, mEq/L	98–106	104		
CO_2, mEq/L	23–30	33		
BUN, mg/dL	10–20	10		
Creatinine, mg/dL	Female: 0.5–1.1	0.8		
Calcium, mg/dL	9.0–10.5	9.0		
Albumin, g/dL	3.5–5.0	2.8		
Total protein, g/dL	6.4–8.3	6.1		
Globulin, g/dL	2.3–3.4	3.3		
A/G ratio	>1.0	0.85		
Bilirubin, total, mg/dL	0.3–1.0	0.9		
ALP, U/L	30–120	110		
ALT, U/L	4–36	38		
AST, U/L	0–35	37		
Osmolality, mOsm/kg H_2O	285–295	280		

Table 5.11: Selected Fasting Values from CBC and Differential Obtained in the ER.

Laboratory Values	Normal Ranges or Values	Susan's Values	Susan's Value (WNL, High or Low)	Implications or Assessment
Hemoglobin, g/dL	Female: 12–16	10		
Hematocrit, %	Female: 37–47	35		
WBC, SI units	5–10	22.6		
Neutrophils, %	55–70	87		
Red blood cell count (RBC), SI units	4.7–6.1	4.2		
Mean corpuscular volume (MCV), fl	80–95	82		
Platelet count × 10^9/L (SI units)	150–400	115		

Table 5.12: Selected Fasting Additional Labs and Vital Signs Obtained in the ER.

Laboratory Values	Normal Ranges or Values	Susan's Values	Susan's Value (WNL, High or Low)	Implications or Assessment
Prealbumin, mg/dL	15–36	11		
CRP, mg/dL	<1.0	34		
HgbA1C, %	<6.0	5.4		
Triglycerides, mg/dL	35–135	105		
Amylase, Somogyi units/dL	60–120	115		
Lipase, units/L	0–110	99		
Lactic acid, mg/dL	Venous: 5–20	6.8 (venous)		
Transferrin, mg/dL	Female: 250–380	397		
Transferrin receptor assay (TIR) mg/L	Female: 1.9–4.4	4,8		
Ferritin, ng/mL	Female: 10–150	8		
TIBC, mcg/dL	250–460	472		
Phosphorus, mg/dL	3.0–4.5	2.7		
Magnesium, mEq/dL	1.3–2.1	1.1		
Temperature, °F	96.4–99.1	103.4		
Blood pressure, mmHg	Systolic <120 Diastolic <80	140/85		
Pulse, beats/minute	60–100	90		
Respirations, breaths/minute	14–20	20		
Pulse oximetry, %	≤95	92		

Hospital Day 2: Susan remained in the Progressive Care unit and reported good pain control with her morphine sulphate PCA. Susan was encouraged to sit in the chair and was assisted in short walks around the nursing station. The nutrition consult was completed with recommendations to start parenteral feeds that afternoon with therapy that was appropriate to prevent refeeding syndrome. Once the TPN was hung, Susan's D5NS IV was dropped to 40 mL/hr. Day 2 medications include prednisone, IV ciprofloxacin, azathioprine, and morphine sulphate PCA. Nursing noted adequate urine output and a soft and nontender abdomen with incisional pain.

Hospital Days 3-4: Susan was transferred to the general surgery floor. She continued to sit in her chair for several hours and was encouraged to ambulate in the hallway several times during the day. On hospital day 4, after reviewing Susan's labs, the interprofessional healthcare team determined that Susan was no longer at risk for refeeding syndrome and the RDN made recommendations to advance the parenteral therapy to meet 100% of Susan's estimated nutritional goals. Once the new TPN was hung, the IVF were discontinued. Nursing continued to report adequate urine output and a soft and nontender abdomen with incisional pain. Medications include prednisone, IV ciprofloxacin, azathioprine, and morphine sulphate PCA.

Table 5.13: BMP, Osmolality, Magnesium, and Phosphorus Obtained on Day 4.

Laboratory Values	Normal Ranges or Values	Susan's Values	Susan's Value (WNL, High or Low)	Implications or Assessment
Glucose, mg/dL	70–110	144		
BUN, mg/dL	10–20	14		
Creatinine, mg/dL	Female: 0.5–1.1	0.8		
Sodium, mEq/L	136–145	139		
Chloride, mEq/L	98–106	102		
Potassium. mEq/L	3.5–5.0	3.8		
CO_2, mmol/L	23–30	26		
Osmolality, mOsm/kg H_2O	285–295	291		
Phosphorus, mg/dL	3.0–4.5	4.1		
Magnesium, mEq/dL	1.3–2.1	2.0		

Hospital Days 5-7: Susan continued to sit in her chair for several hours and continued to ambulate in the hallway several times during the day. She would even venture into the hospital outdoor healing garden to enjoy the sunset. The surgeon wanted to continue full parenteral feeds for at least another seven to ten days due to the status of Susan's abdomen at the time of surgery and the need for nutritional replenishment. He felt this was best with Susan's past medical history. He would allow Susan to suck on some ice chips, but nothing else. A repeat CT scan on hospital day 6 showed no intraabdominal inflammation, blockage or abscesses. On hospital day 7, the surgeon ordered a nutrition consult for home cyclic parenteral feeding recommendations. He wanted to start the cyclic feeds later that night in preparation for discharge later the following day. Nursing continued to report adequate urine output and a soft and nontender abdomen with diminishing incisional pain during this time. Day 5–7 medications include prednisone, IV ciprofloxacin, azathioprine, and morphine sulphate prn.

Table 5.14: Comprehensive Metabolic Panel, A/G Ratio, and Osmolality Obtained on Day 7.

Laboratory Value	Normal Ranges or Values	Susan's Laboratory Values: ER	Susan's Value (WNL, High or Low)	Implications or Assessment
Glucose, mg/dL	70–110	168		
Sodium, mEq/L	136–145	143		
Potassium, mEq/L	3.5–5.0	4.6		
Chloride, mEq/L	98–106	100		
CO2, mEq/L	23–30	26		
BUN, mg/dL	10–20	13		
Creatinine, mg/dL	Female: 0.5–1.1	0.7		
Calcium, mg/dL	9.0–10.5	9.4		
Albumin, g/dL	3.5–5.0	3.4		
Total protein, g/dL	6.4–8.3	6.9		
Globulin, g/dL	2.3–3.4	3.2		
A/G ratio	>1.0	1.06		
Bilirubin, total, mg/dL	0.3–1.0	1.0		
ALP, U/L	30–120	84		
ALT, U/L	4–36	29		
AST, U/L	0–35	24		
Osmolality, mOsm/kg H_2O	285–295	290		

Table 5.15: Selected Values from CBC and Differential Obtained on Day 7.

Laboratory Values	Normal Ranges or Values	Susan's Values	Susan's Value (WNL, High or Low)	Implications or Assessment
Hemoglobin, g/dL	Female: 12–16	14		
Hematocrit, %	Female: 37–47	39		
WBC, SI units	5–10	9.6		
Neutrophils, %	55–70	63		
Platelet count SI units	150–400	264		

Table 5.16: Selected Additional Labs and Vital Signs Obtained on Day 7.

Laboratory Values	Normal Ranges or Values	Susan's Values	Susan's Value (WNL, High or Low)	Implications or Assessment
Prealbumin, mg/dL	15–36	16		
CRP, mg/dL	<1.0	24		
Triglycerides, mg/dL	35–135	115		
Transferrin, mg/dL	Female: 250–380	377		
Transferrin Receptor Assay (TIR) mg/L	Female: 1.9–4.4	4.2		
Ferritin, ng/mL	Female: 10–150	78		
TIBC, mcg/dL	250–460	442		
Phosphorus, mg/dL	3.0–4.5	3.7		
Magnesium, mEq/dL	1.3–2.1	1.9		

Hospital Day 8: Susan tolerated the cyclic parenteral feeds well. Her abdominal pain had diminished and she was frequently seen walking around the nursing station. Susan could continue to take ice chips as desired and all her medications were changed to an oral administration route. She was discharged home on cyclic parenteral feeds. Susan had a follow-up appointment with her physician in one week with plans to stop the cyclic parenteral feeds and advance her diet. Discharge medications include ciprofloxacin, azathioprine, and Percocet prn. The prednisone was changed to a lower dose with plans to wean Susan off the prednisone over several days.

Case Evaluation

Prioritize Problems and Identify Interprofessional Care

1. List in order of importance Susan's medical/nutritional concerns on hospital day 2.

2. Review the concerns listed in question 1. Which member of the healthcare team should address each concern and how should the concern be addressed?

3. List in order of importance Susan's medical/nutritional concerns on hospital day 4.

4. Review the concerns listed in question 3. Which member of the healthcare team should address each concern and how should the concern be addressed?

5. List in order of importance Susan's medical/nutritional concerns on hospital day 7.

6. Review the concerns listed in question 5. Which member of the healthcare team should address each concern and how should the concern be addressed?

7. List in order of importance Susan's medical/nutritional concerns once the cyclic parenteral feeds are discontinued and her diet is advanced.

8. Review the concerns listed in question 7. Which member of the healthcare team should address each concern and how should the concern be addressed?

Disease Process and Laboratory Interpretation

9. Describe the differences between Crohn's disease and ulcerative colitis.

10. Are there laboratory values or vital signs above that would be a concern regarding Susan's condition upon her arrival in the ER?

11. Describe three long-term complications associated with Crohn's disease?

12. Why is important that Susan has her ileocecal valve?

13. a. What is refeeding syndrome?

b. What specific labs are altered with refeeding syndrome? How are they altered?

c. What must one do to with regards to nutrition support to prevent refeeding syndrome in patients at risk?

    d. What is your evaluation of Susan's labs on day 2 and day 3 with regards to risk of refeeding syndrome and ability to advance parenteral feeds to meet 100% nutritional needs?

    e. Do you think it is possible to develop refeeding syndrome when taking an exclusive po diet? Explain your reasoning for the high or low risk.

Anthropometric and Nutrition Assessment

14. a. What is your evaluation of Susan's height/weight status upon arrival in the ER?

    b. What is the most likely cause of weight gain reflected in Susan's ER weight?

15. What is Susan's percentage of weight change over the last month? Describe any concerns regarding this weight change.

16. What is Susan's percentage of weight change since diagnosis with Crohn's disease? Describe any concerns regarding this weight change.

17. Would you encourage Susan to gain weight while receiving TPN post-op? Explain.

18. Upon admit to the hospital, can Susan be diagnosed with malnutrition based on the ASPEN/AND guidelines? Explain.

19. You are performing a nutrition focused physical assessment on Susan while she is in the hospital. Describe what you would expect to find in this assessment.

20. What is your general assessment of Susan's typical dietary intake? Do you feel she is consuming adequate, excessive or deficient energy and protein based on her nutritional requirements in general and in the weeks prior to her admit?

21. Can you determine if Susan may have a diet deficient in micronutrients based on her current typical dietary intake? Explain.

22. Can you determine if Susan may have nutritional deficiencies in micronutrients based on her medical and surgical history? Explain.

23. **a.** Calculate Susan's total energy and protein requirements for her parenteral feedings on day 2. Justify your reasoning for method to determine needs.

b. Calculate Susan's total energy and protein requirements for her parenteral feedings on day 4. Justify your reasoning for method to determine needs.

c. Calculate Susan's total energy and protein requirements once her diet can be advanced as an outpatient. Justify your reasoning for method to determine needs.

Medications

24. Describe the main function of prednisone. Describe possible adverse side effects or drug–nutrient interactions with this medication.

25. Describe the main function of ciprofloxacin. Describe possible adverse side effects or drug–nutrient interactions with this medication.

26. Describe the main function of azathioprine. Describe possible adverse side effects or drug–nutrient interactions with this medication.

27. Describe the main function of morphine. Describe possible adverse side effects or drug–nutrient interactions with this medication.

Nutrition Intervention and Recommendations

28. **a.** What is your initial 2 in 1 parenteral feeding recommendation for Susan on day 2? Refer to energy and protein needs cited in question 23a. Provide recommendations by citing total grams of protein and CHO/day; grams/kg protein; glucose infusion rate (GIR); TPN goal rate/hr.

    b. Cite IVFE total volume infused; grams fat/kg and IVFE infusion rate and duration.

    c. Cite total energy from TPN and IVFE; % protein kcal, % CHO kcal and % fat kcal; total volume infused.

29. **a.** What is your revised 2 in 1 parenteral feeding recommendation for Susan on day 4? Refer to energy and protein needs cited in question 23b. Provide recommendations by citing total grams of protein and CHO/day; grams/kg protein; GIR; TPN goal rate/hr.

    b. Cite IVFE total volume infused; grams fat/kg and IVFE infusion rate and duration.

c. Cite total energy from TPN and IVFE; % protein kcal, % CHO kcal, and % fat kcal; total volume infused.

27. a. What is your cyclic 2 in 1 parenteral feeding recommendation for Susan on day 7? Refer to energy and protein needs cited in question 23b. Provide recommendations by citing total grams of protein and CHO/day; grams/kg protein; GIR; TPN goal rate/hr and specific time frame the cyclic TPN will run.

b. Cite IVFE total volume infused; grams fat/kg and IVFE infusion rate and duration.

c. Cite total energy from TPN and IVFE; % protein kcal, % CHO kcal and % fat kcal; total volume infused.

28. Cite your nutrition recommendations for Susan once her diet is advanced. Specifically, what dietary modifications would you recommend?

Monitoring and Evaluation; Patient Follow-Up

29. a. A. Once Susan is advanced to full parenteral feeds on day 4, how often should Susan's tolerance and response to her parenteral feedings be evaluated?

b. Explain how you would evaluate tolerance to parenteral feeds and labs you would suggest obtaining.

30. a. A. Once Susan is advanced to cyclic parenteral feeds on day 7, how often should Susan's tolerance and response to her parenteral feedings be evaluated?

b. Explain how you would evaluate tolerance to cyclic parenteral feeds and labs you would suggest obtaining.

Academy of Nutrition and Dietetics (AND) Medical Nutrition Therapy (MNT) Guidelines and Documentation for Dietitians.

Nutrition Diagnosis Utilizing the PES statements:

a. Day 2—Initial consult

b. Day 4—Risk of refeeding resolved

c. Day 7—Change to cyclic parenteral feeds

d. Diet advancement as an outpatient

Nutrition Intervention and Goals utilizing AND terminology:

a. Day 2—Initial consult

b. Day 4—Risk of refeeding resolved

c. Day 7—Change to cyclic parenteral feeds

d. Diet advancement as an outpatient

Nutrition Monitoring and Evaluation utilizing AND terminology:

a. Day 2—Initial consult

b. Day 4—Risk of refeeding resolved

c. Day 7—Change to cyclic parenteral feeds

d. Diet advancement as an outpatient

REFERENCE LIST

Ayers, Phil, et al. "Acid-Base Disorders: Learning the Basics." *Nutrition in Clinical Practice*, vol. 30, 2015, pp. 14–20.

Barber, Jacqueline R., and Gordon S. Sacks. "Parenteral Nutrition Formulations." *ASPEN Adult Nutrition Support Core Curriculum*, edited by Charles M. Mueller, 2nd ed., American Society of Parenteral and Enteral Nutrition, 2012, pp. 245–64.

Charney, Pamela. "The Nutrition Care Process." *Pocket Guide to Nutrition Assessment*, edited by Pamela Charney, and Ainsley Malone, 3rd ed., Academy of Nutrition and Dietetics, 2016, pp. 1–14.

Cresi, Gail, and Arlene Escero. "Medical Nutrition Therapy for Lower Gastrointestinal Tract Disorders." *Krause's Food and the Nutrition Care Process*, edited by Kathleen Mahn and Janice L. Raymond, 14th ed., Elsevier, 2017, pp. 525–59.

Crohn's and Colitis Foundation of America. http://www.ccfa.org/.

Franz, Davis, et al. "Gastrointestinal Disease." *ASPEN Adult Nutrition Support Core Curriculum*, edited by Charles M. Mueller, 2nd ed., American Society of Parenteral and Enteral Nutrition, 2012, pp. 426–53.

Ireton-Jones, Carol, and Mary Kristofak Russell. "Food and Nutrient Delivery: Nutrition Support." *Krause's Food and the Nutrition Care Process*, edited by Kathleen Mahn and Janice L. Raymond, 14th ed., Elsevier, 2017, pp. 209–26.

Jenson, Gordon L., et al. "Nutrition Screening and Assessment." *ASPEN Adult Nutrition Support Core Curriculum*, edited by Charles M. Mueller, 2nd ed., American Society of Parenteral and Enteral Nutrition, 2012, pp. 155–69.

Jones, Keaton I., et al. "Simple Psoas Cross-Sectional Area Measurement is a Quick and Easy Method to Assess Sarcopenia and Predicts Major Surgical Complications." *Colorectal Disease*, vol. 17, no. 1, Jan. 2015, pp. 20–26.

Kumpf, Vanessa J., and Jane Gervasio. "Complications of Parenteral Nutrition." *ASPEN Adult Nutrition Support Core Curriculum*, edited by Charles M. Mueller, 2nd ed., American Society of Parenteral and Enteral Nutrition, 2012, pp. 284–97.

Kuroki, Lindsay M., et al. "Pre-operative Assessment of Muscle Mass to Predict Surgical Complications and Prognosis in Patients with Endometrial Cancer." *Annals of Surgical Oncology*, vol. 22, no. 3, Mar. 2015, pp. 972–79.

Langley, Ginger, and Sharla Tajchman. "Fluids, Electrolytes and Acid-Base Disorders." *ASPEN Adult Nutrition Support Core Curriculum,* edited by Charles M. Mueller, 2nd ed., American Society of Parenteral and Enteral Nutrition, 2012, pp. 98–120.

Malone, Ainsley, and Cynthia Hamilton. "The Academy of Nutrition and Dietetics/The American Society for Parenteral and Enteral Nutrition Consensus Malnutrition Characteristics: Application in Practice." *Nutrition in Clinical Practice,* vol. 28, 2013, pp. 639–50.

Merck Manual Professional Version. http://www.merckmanuals.com/professional/.

Mirtallo, Jay M., and Patel Meera. "Overview of Parenteral Nutrition." *ASPEN Adult Nutrition Support Core Curriculum*, edited by Charles M. Mueller, 2nd ed., American Society of Parenteral and Enteral Nutrition, 2012, pp. 234–44.

Nelms, Marcia. "Diseases of the Lower Gastrointestinal Tract." *Nutrition Therapy and Pathophysiology*, edited by Marcia Nahikian-Nelms, 3rd ed., Wadsworth, Cengage Learning, 2016.

____. "Enteral and Parenteral Nutrition Support." *Nutrition Therapy and Pathophysiology*, edited by Marcia Nahikian-Nelms, 3rd ed., Wadsworth, Cengage Learning, 2016, pp. 88–114.

____. "Metabolic Stress and the Critically Ill." *Nutrition Therapy and Pathophysiology*, edited by Marcia Nahikian-Nelms, 3rd ed., Wadsworth, Cengage Learning, 2016.

Nelms, Marcia, and Diane Habash. "Nutrition Assessment: Foundation of the Nutrition Care Process." *Nutrition Therapy and Pathophysiology*, edited by Marcia Nahikian-Nelms, 3rd ed., Wadsworth, Cengage Learning, 2016.

Pagana, Kathleen Deska, and Timothy James Pagana. *Mosby's Manual of Diagnostic and Laboratory Tests*. Mosby/Elsevier, 2014.

Peterson, Sarah J. "Nutrition Focused Physical Assessment." *Pocket Guide to Nutrition Assessment*, edited by Pamela Charney and Ainsley Malone, 3rd ed., Academy of Nutrition and Dietetics, 2016, pp. 76–102.

Teigen, Levi M., et al. "The Use of Technology for Estimating Body Composition: Strengths and Weaknesses of Common Modalities in a Clinical Setting." *Nutrition in Clinical Practice*, vol. 32, no. 1, Feb. 2017, pp. 20–29.

van Leeuwen, Anne, and Mickey Lynn Bladh. *Davis's Comprehensive Handbook of Laboratory & Diagnostic Tests with Nursing Implications*, 6th ed., F. A. Davis, 2015.

Wojda, Thomas R., et al. "Ultrasound and Computed Tomography Imaging Technologies for Nutrition Assessment in Surgical and Critical Care Patient Populations." *Current Surgery Reports*, vol. 3, no. 8, 2015.

CHAPTER **6**

Neurological Concerns

- -

Case Study: Inpatient/Outpatient with Hypertension, Transient Ischemic Attack Including Long-Term Follow-Up

Case-Specific Learning Objectives

- ✓ Assess risk of developing complications associated with hypertension (HTN)
- ✓ Evaluate techniques for the diagnosis of dysphagia.
- ✓ Plan an appropriate diet using the National Dysphagia Dietary principles.
- ✓ Plan an appropriate diet using the DASH diet.

Our Patient: Norman C. is a sixty-four-year-old African American semiretired plumber. Two years ago, he decreased his work schedule to two 10-hour days per week. He is married and has three grown children and four grandchildren. Norman's wife is a homemaker who has been taking care of their two youngest grandchildren, a two-year-old boy and four-year-old girl for the past year. Norman enjoys spending time in the park with his grandchildren. He walks 2 miles or rides his bike 5 miles each morning he does not report to his job. Norman smoked for thirty years before quitting fifteen years ago. His parents passed away from cardiovascular disease when they were both in their early seventies. Norman has one sister who has salt sensitivity and HTN.

Medical and Surgical History: Norman had an appendectomy when he was ten. He suffered broken ribs in a car accident when he was eighteen. Sixteen years ago, Norman was diagnosed with HTN associated with salt sensitivity. He was placed on medications to control his blood pressure. He received education regarding lowering his salt intake; diet modifications to promote weight loss and decreasing the risk of complications associated with HTN. Norman reports concern for long-term complications with this diagnosis and overall very good compliance to his DASH diet, exercise, and medication regime.

Norman sprained his ankle two months ago when playing in the park with his grandchildren. Since that time, Norman has been unable to take his regular walks or ride his bike. He watches movies, reads books, or plays board games with his grandchildren since his injury. He again cites compliance with his diet and medication regime; however, he has gained 6 pounds since he sprained his ankle.

Home Medications: Norman was prescribed furosemide and metoprolol to control his blood pressure. Medication doses have been adjusted over the years to allow excellent blood pressure control.

History of Current Illness: Early one morning approximately one month ago, Norman's wife heard a thud in the bedroom after Norman awoke. She was in the kitchen making breakfast of eggbeaters, toast, jam, orange juice, and coffee. When she arrived in the bedroom, Norman was lying on the ground next to the bed and he appeared confused. When she asked Norman what happened, he was unable to respond and the left side of his face appeared "droopy." She immediately called 911 and the paramedics transported Norman to the local hospital.

Emergency Room and Day 1 Events: Upon arrival, Norman appeared confused and when he tried to speak, his language was slurred and incomprehensible. He was unable to lift his left arm above his head. Norman presented with high blood pressure and was given IV labetalol to successfully lower his blood pressure. The emergency room (ER) physician suspected a stroke and sent Norman directly to radiology for magnetic resonance imaging (MRI) of the brain. He also underwent an electroencephalogram (EEG), an evoked response test, and a blood flow test. The testing determined Norman's stroke was caused by a blockage in the right carotid artery. It was determined that Norman presented as a level 2 according to the National Institutes of Health (NIH) Health Stroke Scale. Intravenous tissue plasminogen activator (tPA) therapy was initiated and Norman was admitted to the Progressive Care Unit. Admit orders indicated Norman would be confined to bed and npo for his first twenty-four hours in the hospital.

Anthropometrics per Wife

Height: 5 feet 10 inches; weight at doctor appointment one month earlier: 190 pounds

Table 6.1: Fasting Lipid Panel Obtained in the ER.

Laboratory Values	Normal Ranges or Values	Norman's Values	Norman's Value (WNL, High or Low)	Implications or Assessment
Triglycerides, mg/dL	Male: 40–160	190		
HDL cholesterol, mg/dL	Male: >45	43		
LDL cholesterol, mg/dL	60–180	192		
Total cholesterol, mg/dL	<200	235		

Table 6.2: Fasting BMP Obtained in ER.

Laboratory Values	Normal Ranges or Values	Norman's Values	Norman's Value (WNL, High or Low)	Implications or Assessment
Glucose, mg/dL	70–110	88		
BUN, mg/dL	10–20	12		
Creatinine, mg/dL	Male: 0.6–1.2	0.8		
Sodium mEq/L	136–145	144		
Chloride, mEq/L	98–106	100		
Potassium, mEq/L	3.5–5.0	3.2		
CO_2, mEq/L	23–30	28		
Osmolality, mOsm/Kg H_2O	285–295	291		

Table 6.3: Fasting Selected Additional Lab Values and Vital Signs Obtained in the ER.

Laboratory Values or Vital Signs	Normal Ranges or Values	Norman's Values	Norman's Value (WNL, High or Low)	Implications or Assessment
Hemoglobin, g/dL	Male: 14–18	15		
Hematocrit, %	Male: 42–52	46		
WBC, SI units	5–10	9.2		
Calcium, mg/dL	9.0–10.5	9.9		
Albumin, g/d	3.5–5.0	4.6		
Prealbumin, mg/dL	15–36	15		
Crp, mg/dL	<1.0	8.1		
HgbA1C, %	<6.0	5.9		
Cardiac troponins, ng/mL	<0.1	0.0		
Ischemia modified albumin, IU/mL	<85	14		
Temperature, °F	96.4–99.1	97.9		
Blood pressure, mmHg	Systolic <120 Diastolic <80	195/155, decreasing to 165/105 after IV labetalol		
Pulse, beats/minute	60–100	95		

(Continued)

Table 6.3 (*continued*)

Laboratory Values or Vital Signs	Normal Ranges or Values	Norman's Values	Norman's Value (WNL, High or Low)	Implications or Assessment
Respirations: breaths/minute	14–20	20		
Pulse oximetry, %	≤95	99		
Body weight: ER Bedscale		94.0 kg		

Hospital Days 2-4: Norman remained in the hospital for a total of four days. During this time, his blood pressure was monitored and controlled with medications. On the second hospital day, physical defects resulting from the stroke were assessed and appropriate rehabilitative therapy was initiated. Physical and Occupational therapy was initiated to assist with the diminished function and weakness in the left side of Norman's body. Norman was not able to speak legibly for the first two days he was in the hospital. His speech was slurred and rarely understandable. A swallow evaluation was ordered on hospital day 2 and it was determined that Norman had a rating of 2 on the Dysphagia Severity Scale. A National Dysphagia Diet 2 or mechanically altered diet with nectar-like fluids was ordered. Norman would be discharged to a rehabilitation facility on this diet.

Typical Dietary Intake per Wife

Breakfast: Norman usually ate the same breakfast of eggbeaters or low-sodium ham, toast, jam, orange juice, and coffee.

Lunch: Norman eats some sort of meat sandwich (chicken, turkey, or roast beef with cheese, veggies, and mayonnaise) or pasta with meat or cheese sauce. He has fast food once per week with his grandchildren. Norman and the grandchildren always have a cookie, ice cream, or fresh fruit for dessert. Norman drinks fruit juice or water with his lunch and always has a glass of 1% milk with his cookie.

Dinner: Norman would consume baked or grilled meat; usually chicken, pork chops, steak or fish plus potatoes, rice or pasta, and a large mixed veggie salad with assorted dressings or a large portion of steamed vegetables. Norman's wife describes his typical portions as "large." Norman occasionally has a glass of red wine with dinner and always has a glass of water.

Rehabilitation Course: Norman remained in a rehabilitation facility near his home for 3½ weeks after discharge from the hospital. His wife would visit him daily at mealtimes. His children and grandchildren visited him a couple times each week at night and each weekend. Norman was very motivated with his therapy and was able to demonstrate progress each day.

When Norman was discharged, he still had some weakness in his left arm and leg. He was able to safely walk with a cane. He continued to have some issues advancing his diet so he remained on the National Dysphagia Diet 2; mechanically altered diet with nectar-like fluids. He was advised to continue with his prior low sodium and DASH modifications as they fit into this dysphagia diet. Prescribed medications for home include furosemide, metoprolol, and warfarin.

Norman's Long-Term Progress: Norman continued to receive outpatient therapy for physical and nutritional concerns for the next six months. After this time, all of his deficits had resolved. His doctor encouraged Norman to continue with a routine exercise program and he was advanced to a regular low-sodium DASH diet.

— — — — — — — — — — — — — — — — — —

Case Evaluation

Prioritize Problems and Identify Interprofessional Care

1. List in order of importance Norman's medical/nutritional concerns on hospital day 2.

   1. Diminished function and weakness in left side of his body
   2. Dysphagia Diet
   3. slurred speach, rarely understandable

2. Review the concerns listed in question 1. Which member of the health-care team should address each concern and how should the concern be addressed?

   • Doctors are assessing affects of stroke
   • physical / occupational Therapists for diminished function
   • Dietician & speech Pathologist for Dysphagia & slurred speech.
   • RD continues to monitor hypertension & salt sensitivity.

Disease Process and Laboratory Interpretation

3. Are there laboratory values or vital signs above that would be a concern regarding to Norman's condition upon admit to the hospital?

4. Norman was at risk for having a transient ischemic attack (TIA). Describe his risk factors.

5. Describe three chronic medical complications associated with HTN?

6. After Norman had his stroke, he was left with some temporary physical deficits. Describe these deficits and how they will affect his lifestyle and recovery.

Anthropometric and Nutrition Assessment

7. What is your evaluation of Norman's height/weight status upon admit to the ER?

   70 inches

   BMI = 27.32 overweight

8. What is Norman's percentage of weight change over the last month prior to his stroke? Describe any concerns regarding this weight change.

   Gained 6 lbs before stroke

   3.2% increase of weight gain

9. Would you encourage Norman to lose weight upon discharge from the rehab facility? Explain.

10. Upon admit to the hospital, can Norman be diagnosed with malnutrition based on the ASPEN/AND guidelines? Explain.

11. Calculate Norman's total energy and protein requirements while in the hospital. Justify your reasoning for method to determine needs.

12. What is your general assessment of Norman's typical dietary intake? Do you feel that he is consuming adequate, excessive, or deficient energy and protein based on his nutritional requirements?

13. Can you determine if Norman may have a diet deficient in micronutrients based on his typical dietary intake? Explain.

14. Can you determine if Norman may have been compliant with the DASH diet based on his typical dietary intake? Explain.

Medications

15. Describe the main functions of furosemide and metoprolol. Describe possible adverse side effects or drug–nutrient interactions with these medications.

16. Could Norman take an alternative diuretic to prevent hypokalemia? Explain.

17. Describe the main function of the tPA therapy including adverse side effects that may be associated with this therapy.

18. Norman is discharged from the rehabilitation facility on warfarin. What are the specific nutritional concerns associated with this medication?

Nutrition Intervention and Recommendations

19. Could dietary modifications alleviate hypokalemia? Describe specific diet therapy/foods to increase potassium intake.

20. Describe the National Dysphagia Diet 1. What are the unique properties of this diet and why is it prescribed?

    Purueed Diet - Smoothe, no lumps

21. Describe the National Dysphagia Diet 2. What are the unique properties of this diet and why is it prescribed?

    Soft foods,

22. Describe the National Dysphagia Diet 3. What are the unique properties of this diet and why is it prescribed?

23. **a.** Describe how dysphagia is diagnosed and the Dysphagia Severity Scale.

b. How would Norman's nutritional recommendations change if he had been diagnosed with a rating of 6?

feeding tube (severe)

c. How would Norman's nutritional recommendations change if he had been diagnosed with a rating of 4?

moderate - needs observation

24. Evaluate the foods from Norman's typical dietary intake. Identify the foods that might not be tolerated or require modification on the prescribed dysphagia, DASH, and low-sodium diets noted in each column heading. For each food identified as a potential problem, provide an appropriate substitute.

Food or Beverage	OK on National Dysphagia Diet 1? If Not, Make an Appropriate Substitute	OK on National Dysphagia Diet 2? If Not, Make an Appropriate Substitute	OK on National Dysphagia Diet 3? If Not, Make an Appropriate Substitute	OK on Low-Sodium or DASH Diet?
Breakfast				
cream of wheat				
pureed banana				
brown sugar				
milk				
Lunch				
Dinner				
chicken pot pie				

Food or Beverage	OK on National Dysphagia Diet 1? If Not, Make an Appropriate Substitute	OK on National Dysphagia Diet 2? If Not, Make an Appropriate Substitute	OK on National Dysphagia Diet 3? If Not, Make an Appropriate Substitute	OK on Low-Sodium or DASH Diet?
Additional Snacks				

Monitoring and Evaluation: Patient Follow-Up

25. Please describe a desired nutritional care follow-up schedule. What should be addressed at follow-up appointments.

26. What specific dietary questions would you ask Norman in a follow-up to see if he understands the prescribed dysphagia diets?

27. What questions would you include in question 26 to make sure that Norman is compliant with low-sodium/DASH modifications?

28. What indicators need to be present to allow Norman to advance from the National Dysphagia diets at each stage?
    a. Advance from stages 1 to 2

    b. Advance from stages 2 to 3

    c. Advance beyond stage 3 to a regular diet?

29. Do you feel Norman will be compliant with his diet upon discharge? Explain.

Academy of Nutrition and Dietetics (AND) Medical Nutrition Therapy (MNT) Guidelines and Documentation for Dietitians

Nutrition Diagnosis Utilizing the PES statements:

In the hospital:

After discharge home from rehabilitation facility:

Nutrition Intervention and Goals Utilizing AND Terminology:

In the hospital:

After discharge home from rehabilitation facility:

Nutrition Monitoring and Evaluation Utilizing AND Terminology:

In the hospital:

After discharge home from rehabilitation facility:

REFERENCE LIST

American Heart Association, http://www.heart.org/.

American Stroke Association, http://www.stroke.org/.

Charney, Pamela. "The Nutrition Care Process." *Pocket Guide to Nutrition Assessment*, edited by Pamela Charney and Ainsley Malone, 3rd ed., Academy of Nutrition and Dietetics, 2016, pp. 1–14.

Corrigan, Mandy L., et al. "Nutrition in the Stroke Patient." *Nutrition in Clinical Practice,* vol. 26, no. 3, 2011, pp. 225–45.

Irwin, Kathy, and Melissa Hansen-Petrik. "Diseases and Disorders of the Neurological System." *Nutrition Therapy and Pathophysiology*, edited by Marcia Nahikian-Nelms, 3rd ed., Wadsworth, Cengage Learning, 2016.

Kertscher, Berit, et al. "Bedside Screening to Detect Oropharyngeal Dysphagia in Patients with Neurological Disorders: An Updated Systematic Review." *Dysphagia*, vol. 29, 2014, pp. 204–12.

Malone, Ainsley, and Carol Hamilton. "The Academy of Nutrition and Dietetics/The American Society for Parenteral and Enteral Nutrition Consensus Malnutrition Characteristics: Application in Practice." *Nutrition in Clinical Practice,* vol. 28, 2013, pp. 639–50.

Martino, Rosemary, et al. "A Systematic Review of Current Clinical and Instrumental Swallowing Assessment Methods." *Current Physical Medicine and Rehabilitation Reports,* vol. 1, 2013, pp. 267–69.

Merck Manual Professional Version, http://www.merckmanuals.com/professional/nutritional-disorders/nutrition,-c-,-general-considerations/nutrient-drug-interactions.

Nelms, Marcia, and Diane Habash. "Nutrition Assessment: Foundation of the Nutrition Care Process." *Nutrition Therapy and Pathophysiology*, edited by Marcia Nahikian-Nelms, 3rd ed., Wadsworth, Cengage Learning, 2016.

Pagana, Kathleen Deska, and Timothy James Pagana. *Mosby's Manual of Diagnostic and Laboratory Tests*. Mosby/Elsevier, 2014.

Peterson, Sarah J. "Nutrition Focused Physical Assessment." *Pocket Guide to Nutrition Assessment*, edited by Pamela Charney and Ainsley Malone, 3rd ed., Academy of Nutrition and Dietetics, 2016, pp. 76–102.

Pujol, Thomas, et al. "Diseases of the Cardiovascular System." *Nutrition Therapy and Pathophysiology*, edited by Marcia Nahikian-Nelms, 3rd ed., Wadsworth, Cengage Learning, 2016.

Roberts, Susan. "Food and Nutrition Related History." *Pocket Guide to Nutrition Assessment*, edited by Pamela Charney and Ainsley Malone, 3rd ed., Academy of Nutrition and Dietetics, 2016, pp. 34–49.

Ruf, Kathryn., et al. "Nutrition in Neurologic impairment." *ASPEN Adult Nutrition Support Core Curriculum*, edited by Charles M. Mueller, 2nd ed., American Society of Parenteral and Enteral Nutrition, 2012, pp. 363–76.

Umay, Ebru K., et al. "Evaluation of Dysphagia in Early Stroke Patients by Bedside, Endoscopic, and Electrophysiological Methods." *Dysphagia,* vol. 28, 2013, pp. 395–403.

Van, Leeuwen Anne, and Mickey Lynn Bladh. *Davis's Comprehensive Handbook of Laboratory and Diagnostic Tests with Nursing Implications*. 6th ed., F. A. Davis, 2015.

Case Study: Parkinson's Disease

Case-Specific Learning Objectives

- ✓ Plan calorie and nutrient dense nutrition therapy.
- ✓ Assess specific drug–nutrient interactions.

Our Patient: Alex S. is a seventy-seven-year-old retired engineer. He retired at the age of sixty five and has led a very active life since then. After retiring, he traveled all over the world with his wife prior to her passing away from cancer two years ago. He golfed four days per week until he was diagnosed with Parkinson's disease five years ago. This diagnosis was a huge shock to Alex. His wife reported soon after diagnosis that Alex started to withdraw and slow down. Alex stopped golfing two years ago. Alex still lives in the home where his children were raised. His children are concerned about Alex living alone and his ability to care for his aging home. Alex has three children and three grandchildren. Alex enjoys spending time with his teenage grandchildren and enjoys watching their school and sporting events, going out to eat or going to the movies with them. Over the past year, he has been going with another retired engineer to a local casino.

Medical and Surgical History: Alex experienced typical childhood illnesses. He broke his leg while skiing when he was in high school and broke his arm while skiing when he was in college. Both injuries required surgical repair. Alex had a few precancerous moles removed ten years ago and had a precancerous polyp removed from his colon three years ago. Currently his Parkinson's disease has progressed to the point of Alex having an unsteady gait and difficulty chewing. His children took Alex's car away one year ago. His daughter or daughters in laws have been preparing meals for Alex as they are concerned about his safety in the kitchen.

Home Medications: Daily multivitamin, levodopa, and carbidopa.

History of Current Illness: Alex is being seen by his doctor for a routine six-month weight check and follow-up. He reports continued fatigue, taking two naps each day and difficulty with activities of daily living. He is frustrated that his children will no longer let him drive his car. He finds it difficult to stand for any period of time before becoming unsteady on his feet. Alex reports his daughter or daughter in laws bring him prepared meals and groceries each week. He does not like what they have been bringing him lately so he is not eating much, however, reported he eats "enough" when the doctor inquired further. Alex reports that it is harder for him to prepare meals for himself due to his Parkinson's symptoms. Yesterday morning, he spilled a half gallon of milk when trying to pour himself a glass. He left the spilled milk on the floor until his daughter-in-law and teenage grandson arrived to clean it up, later that afternoon. Alex denies any pain or discomfort. He states his appetite is "ok" if his family would bring him the "right foods." Alex's doctor noticed that Alex appeared to smell like he had not taken a shower or bath in several days; he had a general unkempt appearance and his shirt had several food stains on it. Alex told the doctor that he took the bus to this appointment because his daughter has been "too nosey" about his appointments and health.

Routine Six-Month Check Doctor's Appointment

Height: 5 feet 10 inches; weight: 145 pounds

Weight six months ago: 164 pounds

Weight one year ago: 175 pounds

Hand grip strength using dynamometer: Below average for age

Temperature, °F: 98.8

Blood pressure, mmHg: 125/70

Pulse, beats/minute: 80

Respirations: breaths/minute: 18

Pulse oximetry, %: 98%

Physical assessment: No edema; general pallor noted by MD.

Table 6.4: Fasting BMP Obtained Two Weeks Prior to Alex's Routine Follow-Up Doctor's Appointment.

Laboratory Values	Normal Ranges or Values	Alex's Values	Alex's Value (WNL, High or Low)	Implications or Assessment
Glucose, mg/dL	70–110	85		
BUN, mg/dL	10–20	18		
Creatinine, mg/dL	Male: 0.6–1.2	0.8		
Sodium mEq/L	136–145	140		
Chloride, mEq/L	98–106	101		
Potassium, mEq/L	3.5–5.0	4.2		
CO_2, mEq/L	23–30	28		
Osmolality, mOsm/Kg H_2O	285–295	290		

Table 6.5: Fasting Selected Additional Lab Values Obtained Two Weeks Prior to Alex's Routine Follow-Up Doctor's Appointment.

Laboratory Values or Vital Sign s	Normal Ranges or Values	Alex's Values	Alex's Value (WNL, High or Low)	Implications or Assessment
Hemoglobin, g/dL	Male: 14–18	12		
Hematocrit, %	Male: 42–52	39		
Transferrin, mg/dL	Male: 215–365	392		
Transferrin receptor assay (TIR), mg/L	Male: 2–5.0	5.6		
Ferritin, ng/mL	Male: 12–300	28		
TIBC, mcg/dL	250–460	477		
Albumin, g/d	3.5–5.0	3.3		
Prealbumin, mg/dL	15–36	15		
HgbA1C, %	<6.0	5.0		

Case Evaluation

Prioritize Problems and Identify Interprofessional Care

1. List in order of importance Alex's medical/nutritional concerns.

2. Review the concerns listed in question 1. Which member of the health-care team should address each concern and how should the concern be addressed?

Disease Process and Laboratory Interpretation

3. What are the diagnostic criteria for determining if one has Parkinson's disease? Explain and describe.

4. Are there laboratory values or vital signs above that would be a concern regarding to Alex's condition? Explain.

Anthropometric and Nutrition Assessment

5. What is your evaluation of Alex's height/weight status at his most recent doctor's appointment?

6. What percentage of body weight has Alex lost over the past six months? What is the significance of this weight loss?

7. What is the percentage of body weight has Alex lost over the past year? What is the significance of this weight loss?

8. **a.** Can Alex' be diagnosed with malnutrition based on the ASPEN/AND guidelines? Explain.

9. **a.** Describe two to three chronic nutritional concerns that may be associated with Parkinson's disease? Describe how these concerns can lead to a diagnosis of malnutrition.

    b. As Alex's Parkinson's disease progresses, what additional nutritional concerns develop? Explain.

10. Calculate Alex's total energy and protein requirements. Justify your reasoning for method to determine needs.

11. **a.** What is your general assessment of Alex's overall nutritional intake prior to this most recent doctor's appointment?

    b. Describe the barriers or concerns that have caused Alex's overall nutritional intake to decrease?

Medications

12. Describe the main function of levodopa and carbidopa. Describe possible adverse side effects, nutritional concerns or drug–nutrient interactions with these medications.

13. Do you agree with Alex taking a multivitamin each day? Explain

Nutrition Intervention or Recommendations

14. Based on Alex's medical history and current status (weight, labs, etc.), what specific recommendations would you make to increase both the energy and protein content of Alex's diet?

15. What additional recommendations would you make to encourage or allow Alex to consume an adequate nutritional intake? (Hint: think about possible environmental or social concerns too.)

Monitoring and Evaluation: Patient Follow-Up

16. Please describe a desired nutritional care follow-up schedule for Alex. What should be addressed at follow-up appointments.

17. What specific dietary questions would you ask Alex in a follow-up to see if he understands his prescribed nutrition intervention?

Academy of Nutrition and Dietetics (AND) Medical Nutrition Therapy (MNT) Guidelines and Documentation for Dietitians

Nutrition Diagnosis Utilizing the PES Statements:

Nutrition Intervention and Goals Utilizing AND Terminology:

Nutrition Monitoring and Evaluation Utilizing AND Terminology:

REFERENCE LIST

Charney, Pamela. "The Nutrition Care Process." *Pocket Guide to Nutrition Assessment*, edited by Pamela Charney and Ainsley Malone, 3rd ed., Academy of Nutrition and Dietetics, 2016, pp. 1–14.

Irwin, Kathy, and Melissa Hansen-Petrik. "Diseases and Disorders of the Neurological System." *Nutrition Therapy and Pathophysiology*, edited by Marcia Nahikian-Nelms, 3rd ed., Wadsworth, Cengage Learning, 2016.

Malone, Ainsley, and Carol Hamilton. "The Academy of Nutrition and Dietetics/The American Society for Parenteral and Enteral Nutrition Consensus Malnutrition Characteristics: Application in Practice." *Nutrition in Clinical Practice*, vol. 28, 2013, pp. 639–50.

Merck Manual Professional Version, http://www.merckmanuals.com/professional/nutritional-disorders/nutrition,-c-,-general-considerations/nutrient-drug-interactions.

Nelms, Marcia, and Diane Habash. "Nutrition Assessment: Foundation of the Nutrition Care Process." *Nutrition Therapy and Pathophysiology*, edited by Marcia Nahikian-Nelms, 3rd ed., Wadsworth, Cengage Learning, 2016.

Pagana, Kathleen Deska, and Timothy James Pagana. *Mosby's Manual of Diagnostic and Laboratory Tests*. Mosby/Elsevier, 2014.

Parkinson's Disease Foundation, http://www.parkinson.org/.

Peterson, Sarah J. "Nutrition Focused Physical Assessment." *Pocket Guide to Nutrition Assessment*, edited by Pamela Charney and Ainsley Malone, 3rd ed., Academy of Nutrition and Dietetics, 2016, pp. 76–102.

Postuma, Ronald, and Daniela Berg. "MDS Clinical Diagnostic Criteria for Parkinson's Disease (I1.010)." *Neurology*, vol. 86, no. 16, suppl. I1.010, 5 Apr. 2016.

Ruf, Kathryn., et al. "Nutrition in Meurologic Impairment." *ASPEN Adult Nutrition Support Core Curriculum*, edited by Charles M. Mueller, 2nd ed., American Society of Parenteral and Enteral Nutrition, 2012, pp. 363–76.

Tholfson, Lena K., et al. "Development of Excessive Daytime Sleepiness in Early Parkinson Disease." *Neurology,* vol. 85, no. 2, 2015, pp. 162–68.

Van, Leeuwen Anne, and Mickey Lynn Bladh. *Davis's Comprehensive Handbook of Laboratory and Diagnostic Tests with Nursing Implications.* 6th ed., F. A. Davis, 2015.

Zupec-Kania, Beth, and O'Flaherty Therese. "Medical Nutrition Therapy for Neurologic Disorders." *Krause's Food and the Nutrition Care Process*, edited by Kathleen Mahn and Janice L. Raymond, 14th ed., Elsevier, 2017, pp. 813–38.

CHAPTER 7

Oncology and Immunosuppressive Concerns

- -

Case Study: HIV Infection

Case-Specific Learning Objectives

- ✓ Determine appropriate diet therapy for HIV Infection.
- ✓ Identify potential positive or negative effects from herbal consumption.
- ✓ Determine how different stages of disease and treatment can affect nutritional requirements and intake.
- ✓ Evaluate ethnic variations of dietary modifications

Our Patient: Jeff C. is a twenty-eight-year-old male of Asian descent who lives with his significant other; they recently purchased their first home. Jeff and his partner have been in a relationship for eight years. Jeff and his partner are social workers and both work for an agency that addresses issues of elderly individuals. When Jeff was a twenty-year-old college student, his mother passed away from a massive heart attack. He was very close to his mother and became depressed after her death. During this time, he practiced risky behavior and became infected with the HIV virus during his junior year in college. Jeff goes to the gym to either lift weights or swim four to five days per week after work.

Medical and Surgical History: Jeff experienced typical childhood illnesses. He was diagnosed with asthma at age 6 and had no longer required asthma medications by the time he started high school. Jeff had a tonsillectomy when he was eight years old. Jeff's mother had high blood pressure (HTN) and his father has high cholesterol. Jeff has a thirty-year-old sister who is healthy.

Home Medications: MVI. maraviroc, etravirine, and atazanavir.

Quarterly Check-Up: Jeff is 6 feet tall and usually weighs 84.1 kg. Three months ago, at his doctor's appointment, Jeff weighed 82.6 kg. His appetite has been good. Jeff reports the last four weeks have been stressful at work. For the past month, Jeff has overseen reviewing all company policies in preparation for a large corporate review and additional accreditation. He has been working twelve hour shifts and has not been able to go to the gym in the last month. The corporate review is at the end of this week and Jeff felt anxious about taking a couple of hours off work to go to his scheduled quarterly doctor's check-up.

An annual nutrition focused physical exam was performed at this doctor's appointment: The nurse performing the exam noted well-defined muscle in the bilateral temple region; well-defined muscle around the clavicle; curved muscle at the shoulders; no bony prominence at the bilateral scapula; no protrusion of the iliac crest; well-rounded bilateral quadriceps; well-developed muscle bulb in bilateral posterior calf. Jeff's handgrip dynamometer measured 34 kg in his dominant hand.

Typical Dietary Intake: Jeff and his partner typically prepare their meals at home and almost exclusively use organic and whole foods. They rarely buy processed. They love ethnic foods and prepare foods from a variety of regions throughout the world including dishes prepared from Jeff's family recipes. Jeff loves flavorful foods and adds a lot of garlic, a variety of fresh hot peppers and onion in his cooking. Recently, they started to add fresh olive leaves, lemongrass, citrus peel, and licorice root when cooking; the more the better. They even prepare their own condiments; salad dressings, barbeque, and other sauces. They usually go out to eat two to three times per month. For the past two weeks, Jeff skipped breakfast each morning but did stop at Starbucks for a Grande Frappuccino on the way to work. He has been eating fast food for lunch; Taco Bell, McDonalds, Burger King, Raising Cane's, Chipotle, and Panda Express in the past week. Dinner was always after 8:00 p.m. and consisted of pizza and beer, sushi and sake or Mexican food, and margaritas with coworkers. Jeff noted he has felt fatigued all week and attributes this to his work schedule and poor eating habits for the week. He is looking forward to getting back in the kitchen and cooking with his herbs as he feels they give him energy and an overall sense of well-being.

Jeff's doctor spent quite a bit of time discussing his recent lifestyle, weight changes, and increase in blood pressure. Jeff assured his doctor that once this review at work was completed he was going to take a much-needed vacation to relax on a beach and go back to his normal eating and exercise habits. Regardless, Jeff's doctor prescribed captopril for his hypertension, referred Jeff to a Registered Dietitian Nutritionist for nutritional evaluation and recommended a follow-up appointment in one month.

Table 7.1: Selected Vital Signs Obtained at Quarterly Check-Up.

Parameter	Normal Ranges or Values	Jeff's Values	Jeff's Value (WNL, High or Low)	Implications or Assessment
Blood pressure, mmHg	Systolic <130 Diastolic <85	155/100		
Pulse, beats/minute	60–100	85		
Respirations: breaths/minute	14–20	16		
Pulse oximetry, %	≤95	98		

Table 7.2: Quarterly Fasting CMP, BUN/Creatinine, and A/G Ratios and Osmolality Obtained One Week Prior to Check-Up.

Laboratory Values	Normal Ranges or Values	Jeff's Values	Jeff's Value (WNL, High or Low)	Implications or Assessment
Glucose, mg/dL	70–110	93		
Sodium mEq/L	136–145	142		
Potassium, mEq/L	3.5–5.0	4.7		
Chloride, mEq/L	98–106	101		
CO_2, mEq/L	23–30	27		
BUN, mg/dL	10–20	14		
Creatinine, mg/dL	Male: 0.6–1.2	0.8		
BUN/Creatinine ratio	10–20	17.5		
Calcium, mg/dL	9.0–10.5	9.2		
Albumin, g/d	3.5–5.0	3.3		
Total protein, g/dL	6.4–8.3	6.1		
Globulin, g/dL	2.3–3.4	2.5		
Albumin/Globulin ratio	>1.0	1.32		
Bilirubin, total, mg/dL	0.3–1.0	1.0		
ALP, U/L	30–120	120		
ALT, U/L	4–36	35		
AST, U/L	0–35	33		
Osmolality, mOsm/Kg H_2O	285–295	290		

Table 7.3: Quarterly Fasting Selected Values from CBC Obtained One Week Prior to Check-Up.

Laboratory Values	Normal Ranges or Values	Jeff's Values	Jeff's Value (WNL, High or Low)	Implications or Assessment
Hemoglobin, g/dL	Male: 14–18	16		
Hematocrit, %	Male: 42–52	45		
WBC, SI units	5–10	5.1		
Lymphocytes, %	20–40	18		
Monocytes, %	2–8	3		
Neutrophils, %	55–70	58		
Platelet count SI units	150–400	215		

Table 7.4: Quarterly Fasting Selected Additional Labs Obtained One Week Prior to Check-Up.

Laboratory Values	Normal Ranges or Values	Jeff's Values	Jeff's Value (WNL, High or Low)	Implications or Assessment
Prealbumin, mg/dL	15–36	26		
Crp, mg/dL	<1.0	3		
HgbA1C, %	<6.0	5.4		
CD4 cell count, cells/microliter	600–1500	375		
Viral load (PCR), copies/ml	<200	250		
T-lymphocytes, cells/microliter	200–499	245		
LDH, U/L	100–190	215		
Amylase, Somogyi units/dL	60–120	83		
Lipase, units/L	0–110	46		
Transferrin, mg/dL	Male: 215–365	315		
Transferrin receptor assay (TIR) anemia versus chronic disease, mg/L	Male: 2–5.0	3.5		
Ferritin, ng/mL	Male: 12–300	125		
TIBC, mcg/dL	250–460	275		
Phosphorus, mg/dL	3.0–4.5	3.8		

- -

Case Evaluation

Prioritize Problems and Identify Interprofessional Care

1. List in order of importance Jeff's medical/nutritional concerns.

2. Review the concerns listed in question 1. Which member of the health-care team should address each concern and how should the concern be addressed?

Disease Process and Laboratory Interpretation

3. Are there laboratory values or vital signs above that would be a concern regarding to Jeff's condition? Explain.

4. a. Assume Jeff develops progressive immunocompromise and AIDS in the future. Describe additional medical conditions that may develop.

b. Assume Jeff develops progressive immunocompromise and AIDS in the future. Describe potential laboratory and physiologic changes Jeff will experience.

5. Assume Jeff develops AIDS wasting syndrome in the future. Describe this condition.

Anthropometric and Nutrition Assessment

6. What is your evaluation of Jeff's height/weight status?

7. a. What percentage of body weight change has Jeff experienced over the past three months?

    b. What is the cause or significance of this weight change?

8. Can Jeff be diagnosed with malnutrition based on the ASPEN/AND guidelines? Explain.

9. Calculate Jeff's total energy and protein requirements. Justify your reasoning for method to determine needs.

10. What is your general assessment of Jeff's overall nutritional intake prior to this most recent doctor's appointment?

11. Can you determine if Jeff may have a diet deficient in energy, protein, or micronutrients based on his physical exam? Explain.

12. How would energy, protein, and micronutrient needs change if Jeff develops AIDS in the future?

13. Assume Jeff develops AIDS in the future. Describe three different opportunistic conditions that can develop and how they can affect Jeff's nutritional status.

14. What nutritional modifications would be required if Jeff develops complications from AIDS described in 13 above?

Medications

15. Describe the main function of captopril. Describe possible adverse side effects or drug–nutrient interactions with this medication.

16. Describe the main function of maraviroc. Describe possible adverse side effects or drug–nutrient interactions with this medication.

17. Describe the main function of etravirine. Describe possible adverse side effects or drug–nutrient interactions with this medication.

18. Describe the main function of atazanavir. Describe possible adverse side effects or drug–nutrient interactions with this medication.

19. a. Jeff and his partner cook with a variety of herbs. Note any potential benefits from the herbs Jeff incorporates into his meals.

b. Note any potential adverse effects from the herbs Jeff incorporates into his meals.

c. When questioned about amounts of herbs Jeff consumes he notes "a lot." What are your thoughts on adding these items into cooking versus taking these herbs in a pill or supplement form?

Nutrition Intervention and Recommendations

20. a. What conditions are in Jeff's family history that require nutritional habits to be addressed at this appointment?

b. What additional nutrition recommendations would you make regarding Jeff's diet concerning the conditions noted in 20a?

21. Assume Jeff develops diarrhea in the future. Describe specific nutrition recommendations to help alleviate this problem.

22. Assume Jeff develops a decreased appetite in the future. Describe specific nutrition recommendations to help alleviate this problem.

23. Assume Jeff develops oral lesions in the future. Describe specific nutrition recommendations to help alleviate this problem.

Monitoring and Evaluation; Patient Follow-Up

24. Jeff has routine quarterly comprehensive follow-up exams with his doctor. He will be seeing the doctor again in a month due to the new diagnosis of hypertension. Describe a desired nutritional care follow-up schedule for Jeff and what should be addressed at follow-up appointments.

25. What specific dietary questions would you ask Jeff in a follow-up to see if he has any nutritional concerns?

AND Medical Nutrition Therapy (MNT) Guidelines and Documentation for Dietitians

Nutrition Diagnosis Utilizing the PES Statements:

Initial consult

After hypothetical development of oral lesions and diarrhea in the future

Nutrition Intervention and Goals Utilizing AND Terminology:

Initial consult

After hypothetical development of oral lesions and diarrhea in the future

Nutrition Monitoring and Evaluation Utilizing AND Terminology:

Initial consult

After hypothetical development of oral lesions and diarrhea in the future

REFERENCE LIST

Charney, Pamela. "The Nutrition Care Process." *Pocket Guide to Nutrition Assessment*, edited by Pamela Charney and Ainsley Malone, 3rd ed., Academy of Nutrition and Dietetics, 2016, pp. 1–14.

Dong, Kimberly R., and Cindy Mari Imai. "Nutrition Therapy for HIV and AIDS." *Krause's Food and the Nutrition Care Process*, edited by Kathleen Mahn and Janice L. Raymond, 14th ed., Elsevier, 2017, pp. 757–74.

Jenson, Gordon L., et al. "Nutrition Screening and Assessment." *ASPEN Adult Nutrition Support Core Curriculum*, edited by Charles M. Mueller, 2nd ed., American Society of Parenteral and Enteral Nutrition, 2012, pp. 155–69.

Mendelsohn, Robin, and Mark Shattner. "Cancer." *ASPEN Adult Nutrition Support Core Curriculum*, edited by Charles M. Mueller, 2nd ed., American Society of Parenteral and Enteral Nutrition, 2012, pp. 412–25.

Merck Manual Professional Version, http://www.merckmanuals.com/professional/nutritional-disorders/nutrition,-c-,-general-considerations/nutrient-drug-interactions.

Nelms, Marcia, and Diane Habash. "Nutrition Assessment: Foundation of the Nutrition Care Process." *Nutrition Therapy and Pathophysiology*, edited by Marcia Nahikian-Nelms, 3rd ed., Wadsworth, Cengage Learning, 2016.

Pagana, Kathleen Deska, and Timothy James Pagana. *Mosby's Manual of Diagnostic and Laboratory Tests*. Mosby/Elsevier, 2014.

Peterson, Sarah. "Nutrition Focused Physical Assessment." *Pocket Guide to Nutrition Assessment*, edited by Pamela Charney and Ainsley Malone, 3rd ed., Academy of Nutrition and Dietetics, 2016, pp. 76–102.

Sucher, Kathryn. "HIV and AIDS." *Nutrition Therapy and Pathophysiology*, edited by Marcia Nahikian-Nelms, 3rd ed., Wadsworth, Cengage Learning, 2016.

Van Leeuwen, Anne, and Bladh Mickey Lynn. *Davis's Comprehensive Handbook of Laboratory and Diagnostic Tests with Nursing Implications*. 6th ed., F.A. Davis, 2015.

Wasserman, Peter J., et al. *ASPEN Adult Nutrition Support Core Curriculum*. Edited by Charles M. Mueller, 2nd ed., American Society of Parenteral and Enteral Nutrition, 2012, pp. 536–62.

https://www.aids.gov/hiv-aids-basics/just-diagnosed-with-hiv-aids/treatment-options/overview-of-hiv-treatments/.

Case Study: Breast Cancer—Outpatient Nutritional Therapy

Case-Specific Learning Objectives

✓ Determine how different stages of disease and treatment can affect nutritional requirements and intake.

Our Patient: Denise D. is a fifty-two-year-old female elementary school teacher. She is married and has two teenage children; a boy and a girl. Denise comes from a big Italian family and they love to cook and partake in Italian foods, wines, and desserts. Big meals are always part of family gatherings. Denise likes most foods but does have an aversion to legumes, bananas, and kiwi. She will not drink milk, but will consume milk in coffee or cereals. She loves milk products such as ice cream, yogurts, and cheeses. Denise always has fruit and/or veggies with every meal each day.

Medical and Surgical History: Denise has always been healthy. She did suffer from the typical childhood illnesses and broke her wrist ice skating when she was sixteen years old. The wrist fracture required surgical repair. Denise prides herself in taking few medications and had a natural childbirth when delivering both children.

Home Medications: None.

History of Current Illness: Denise was recently diagnosed with stage 2 breast cancer after undergoing her annual screening mammogram. She has a family history of breast cancer as her mother, two aunts, and a sister were diagnosed with breast cancer. All received successful treatment and are in remission. Denise was very upset after her diagnosis of breast cancer and her appetite diminished. Her weight dropped from 148 pounds two weeks prior to the mammogram to 133 pounds at her pre-op appointment with her surgeon, two weeks after the mammogram. After a long discussion with her medical team and family, Denise agreed to undergo a double mastectomy. Denise's doctor ordered pre-op blood work.

Table 7.5: Fasting Comprehensive Metabolic Panel, BUN/Creatinine and A/G Ratios Obtained Pre-Op.

Laboratory Values	Normal Ranges or Values	Denise's Laboratory Values: ER	Denise's Value (WNL, High or Low)	Implications or Assessment
Glucose, mg/dL	70–110	88		
Sodium mEq/L	136–145	142		
Potassium, mEq/L	3.5–5.0	4.6		
Chloride, mEq/L	98–106	100		
CO_2, mEq/L	23–30	28		
BUN, mg/dL	10–20	14		
Creatinine, mg/dL	Female: 0.5–1.1	0.7		
BUN/Creatinine ratio	10–20	20		
Calcium, mg/dL	9.0–10.5	9.2		
Albumin, g/d	3.5–5.0	3.4		
Total protein, g/dL	6.4–8.3	6.2		
Globulin, g/dL	2.3–3.4	2.5		
Albumin/Globulin ratio	>1.0	1.36		
Bilirubin, total, mg/dL	0.3–1.0	0.8		
ALP, U/L	30–120	105		
ALT, U/L	4–36	31		
AST, U/L	0–35	32		

Table 7.6: Selected Values from Fasting Complete Blood Count and Differential Obtained Pre-Op.

Laboratory Values	Normal Ranges or Values	Denise's Laboratory Values: ER	Denise's Value (WNL, High or Low)	Implications or Assessment
Hemoglobin, g/dL	Female: 12–16	12		
Hematocrit, %	Female: 37–47	37		
WBC, SI units	5–10	8.2		
Neutrophils, %	55–70	61		
Lymphocytes, %	20–40	22		
Monocytes, %	2–8	5		
Platelet count SI units	150–400	305		

Hospital and Postoperative Course: Denise underwent a double mastectomy six weeks ago. The surgery was uncomplicated and Denise was hospitalized for three days and then discharged home. Her doctor was concerned about her loss in weight over one month's time preoperatively and had a RDN see Denise in the hospital immediately prior to her discharge. Her physician wanted to minimize additional weight loss prior to the start of chemotherapy. Denise weighed 130 pounds upon discharge from the hospital. The RDN provided Denise with some sound nutritional advice and encouraged her to eat well to minimize the risk of additional weight loss prior to starting her chemotherapy. Furthermore, the RDN provided Denise with basic information regarding possible side effects from her chemotherapy that may produce a further compromise in her nutritional status.

Overall, Denise recovered well from the mastectomy. Denise had a patient-controlled analgesia (PCA) pump to control her pain with morphine sulphate for thirty-six hours post-op. She took Percocet for an additional four days post-op before transitioning to over-the-counter analgesics. Denise resumed normal activity within five days of discharge from the hospital.

Outpatient Chemotherapy Plan: Denise will require four individual days (rounds) of chemotherapy as the remaining treatment for her current condition. Each round (daily treatment) of chemotherapy will be separated by approximately one to two weeks of a rest period where Denise will not receive chemotherapy. She is planning on breast reconstructive surgery in the future. Denise received her first round of chemotherapy sixteen days ago which was exactly two weeks after her double mastectomy. She underwent her second round of chemotherapy two days ago. Denise tolerated her first round of chemotherapy well and complained of some nausea after her second round of treatment two days ago. Her doctor ordered some blood work at the halfway point of her chemotherapy treatments. She had her blood drawn yesterday and results are in Table 7.7.

Outpatient Chemotherapy Medications: IV Taxotre and Cytoxan injections.

Table 7.7: Fasting Comprehensive Metabolic Panel, BUN/Creatinine, and A/G Ratios Obtained After Second Round of Chemotherapy.

Laboratory Values	Normal Ranges or Values	Denise's Laboratory Values: ER	Denise's Value (WNL, High or Low)	Implications or Assessment
Glucose, mg/dL	70–110	75		
Sodium mEq/L	136–145	140		
Potassium, mEq/L	3.5–5.0	3.5		
Chloride, mEq/L	98–106	102		
CO_2, mEq/L	23–30	25		
BUN, mg/dL	10–20	12		
Creatinine, mg/dL	Female: 0.5–1.1	0.6		
BUN/Creatinine ratio	10–20	20		
Calcium, mg/dL	9.0–10.5	8.9		
Albumin, g/d	3.5–5.0	3.1		
Total protein, g/dL	6.4–8.3	6.0		
Globulin, g/dL	2.3–3.4	2.6		
Albumin/Globulin ratio	>1.0	1.19		
Bilirubin, total, mg/dL	0.3–1.0	0.8		
ALP, U/L	30–120	120		
ALT, U/L	4–36	38		
AST, U/L	0–35	35		

Table 7.8: Selected Values from Fasting Complete Blood Count and Differential Obtained After Second Round of Chemotherapy.

Laboratory Values	Normal Ranges or Values	Denise's Laboratory Values: ER	Denise's Value (WNL, High or Low)	Implications or Assessment
Hemoglobin, g/dL	Female: 12–16	13		
Hematocrit, %	Female: 37–47	38		
WBC, SI units	5–10	5.0		
Neutrophils, %	55–70	41		
Lymphocytes, %	20–40	18		
Monocytes, %	2–8	1.4		
Platelet count SI units	150–400	138		

Case Evaluation

Prioritize Problems and Identify Interprofessional Care

1. List in order of importance Denise's medical/nutritional concerns from admit date through her hospital stay.

2. Review the concerns listed in question 1. Which member of the health-care team should address each concern and how should the concern be addressed?

3. List in order of importance Denise's nutritional concerns during her course of chemotherapy treatments.

4. Review the concerns listed in question 3. Which member of the health-care team should address each concern and how should the concern be addressed?

Disease Process and Laboratory Interpretation

5. **a.** Are there laboratory values or vital signs above that would be a concern regarding Denise's condition prior to her mastectomy?

b. Are there laboratory values or vital signs above that would be a concern regarding Denise's condition after her second round of chemotherapy treatments?

c. Assume Denise experiences several adverse gastrointestinal (GI) side effects from the chemotherapy. What changes would you expect to see with regards to Denise's labs after four rounds of chemotherapy? Specifically, what labs would change and how would they change (increase or decrease) and why?

Anthropometric and Nutrition Assessment

6. What is your evaluation of Denise's height/weight status prior to the mammogram?

7. What is the percentage of weight Denise lost from the time prior to her mammogram until her discharge from the hospital? What is the overall impact of this weight change on Denise's nutritional status?

8. What is your evaluation of Denise's height/weight status prior to the start of the chemotherapy?

9. Assume Denise experiences multiple adverse GI side effects from the chemotherapy. What changes would you expect to see with regards to Denise's body weight and composition after four rounds of chemotherapy?

10. Upon admit to the hospital, can Denise be diagnosed with malnutrition based on the ASPEN/AND guidelines? Explain.

11. Is there a reason to expect Denise to have micronutrient deficiencies upon admit to the hospital? Explain.

12. Describe how you would expect to see Denise's total nutritional requirements (energy, protein, and micronutrients) change between the time prior to her diagnosis, immediately post-op from her mastectomy and during her chemotherapy.

13. Calculate Denise's total energy and protein requirements immediately after her mastectomy. Justify your reasoning for method to determine needs.

14. Assume Denise's incisions from her mastectomy have healed. Calculate Denise's total energy and protein requirements during her chemotherapy. Justify your reasoning for method to determine needs.

15. Would you recommend additional micronutrient supplementation while Denise is undergoing chemotherapy? Provide specific details.

Medications

16. Describe the main function of Taxotre. Describe possible adverse side effects or drug-nutrient interactions with this medication.

17. Describe the main function of Cytoxan. Describe possible adverse side effects or drug-nutrient interactions with this medication.

Nutrition Intervention and Recommendations

18. What is your initial nutrition therapy recommendation for Denise on hospital day 2 after her mastectomy?

19. Assume Denise experiences some of the adverse side effects that could impact her nutritional status or oral intake for two to three days after receiving each round of chemotherapy. Her physician ordered a follow-up nutrition consult after the completion of her second round of chemotherapy to address these issues. What recommendations will you make? Ideally, you will provide Denise with two sets of recommendations; one for when she experiences these adverse effects and one for her "good days." Remember to make specific recommendations to minimize the risk of weight loss, body composition changes, and micronutrient deficiencies during this time.

Monitoring and Evaluation; Patient Follow-Up

20. How often should Denise's tolerance and response to her diet be evaluated while she is receiving her chemotherapy? Justify your reasoning.

Academy of Nutrition and Dietetics (AND) Medical Nutrition Therapy (MNT) Guidelines and Documentation for Dietitians

Nutrition Diagnosis Utilizing the PES Statements:

a. Day 2, prior to discharge from the hospital

b. After Denise's second round of chemotherapy

Nutrition Intervention and Goals Utilizing AND Terminology:

a. Day 2, prior to discharge from the hospital

b. After Denise's second round of chemotherapy

Nutrition Monitoring and Evaluation utilizing AND terminology:

a. Day 2, prior to discharge from the hospital

b. After Denise's second round of chemotherapy

REFERENCE LIST

American Cancer Society, http://www.cancer.org/.

Charney, Pamela. "The Nutrition Care Process." *Pocket Guide to Nutrition Assessment*, edited by Pamela Charney and Ainsley Malone, 3rd ed., Academy of Nutrition and Dietetics, 2016, pp. 1–14.

Cohen, Deoborah A., and Kathryn Sucher. "Neoplastic Disease." *Nutrition Therapy and Pathophysiology*, edited by Marcia Nahikian-Nelms, 3rd ed., Wadsworth, Cengage Learning, 2016, pp. 686–710.

Hamilton, Kathryn, and Barbara Grant. "Medical Nutrition Therapy for Cancer Prevention, Therapy and Survivorship." *Krause's Food and the Nutrition Care Process*, edited by Kathleen Mahn and Janice L. Raymond, 14th ed., Elsevier, 2017.

Jenson, Gordon L., et al. "Nutrition Screening and Assessment." *ASPEN Adult Nutrition Support Core Curriculum*, edited by Charles M. Mueller, 2nd ed., American Society of Parenteral and Enteral Nutrition, 2012, pp. 155–69.

Malone, Ainsley, and Cynthia Hamilton. "The Academy of Nutrition and Dietetics/The American Society for Parenteral and Enteral Nutrition Consensus Malnutrition Characteristics: Application in Practice." *Nutrition in Clinical Practice*, vol. 28, 2013, pp. 639–50.

Mendelsohn, Robin, and Mark Shattner. "Cancer." *ASPEN Adult Nutrition Support Core Curriculum*, edited by Charles M. Mueller, 2nd ed., American Society of Parenteral and Enteral Nutrition, 2012, pp. 412–25.

Merck Manual Professional Version, http://www.merckmanuals.com/professional/nutritional-disorders/nutrition,-c-,-general-considerations/nutrient-drug-interactions.

Nelms, Marcia, and Diane Habash. "Nutrition Assessment: Foundation of the Nutrition Care Process." *Nutrition Therapy and Pathophysiology*, edited by Marcia Nahikian-Nelms, 3rd ed., Wadsworth, Cengage Learning, 2016.

Pagana, Kathleen Deska, and Timothy James Pagana. *Mosby's Manual of Diagnostic and Laboratory Tests.* Mosby/Elsevier, 2014.

Peterson, Sarah. "Nutrition Focused Physical Assessment." *Pocket Guide to Nutrition Assessment*, edited by Pamela Charney and Malone Malone, 3rd ed., Academy of Nutrition and Dietetics, 2016, pp. 76–102.

Van Leeuwen, Anne, and Bladh Mickey Lynn. *Davis's Comprehensive Handbook of Laboratory and Diagnostic Tests with Nursing Implications.* 6th ed., F.A. Davis, 2015.

http://www.breastcancer.org/treatment/druglist/cytoxan.

http://www.breastcancer.org/treatment/druglist/taxotere.

Case Study: Ovarian Cancer and Pelvic Radiation Disease

Case-Specific Learning Objectives

✓ Evaluate clinical, laboratory, and dietary information to assess malnutrition.

✓ Determine how different stages of disease and treatment can affect nutritional requirements and intake.

✓ Develop and calculate parenteral nutrition support therapy.

✓ Identify characteristics of and plan feeds for prevention of refeeding syndrome.

✓ Develop Cyclic parenteral nutrition therapy.

Our Patient: Mona G. is a forty-four-year-old female who was diagnosed with stage 2 ovarian cancer nine months ago. She is married and has four children ages nine, twelve, thirteen, and seventeen years. She was employed as a pharmacist until her diagnosis, subsequent cancer treatments and surgery. She has not worked in seven months. Mona's husband is a respiratory therapist. Mona's parents moved in with her family six months ago to help care for Mona and assist with her children. Mona's parents assist with shopping, meal preparation, housecleaning, and chauffeuring her children to various activities. Mona is 5 feet 5 inches tall. She weighed 145 pounds prior to her diagnosis of ovarian cancer and weighed 128 pounds one month after her surgery.

Medical and Surgical History: Mona suffered from the normal childhood illnesses. She was diagnosed with asthma when she was six and had stopped taking all asthma medications by the age of twelve. Mona still suffers from seasonal allergies, but these episodes do not cause adverse symptoms related to asthma. Three of Mona's pregnancies and deliveries were uncomplicated. Mona developed borderline gestational diabetes when she was pregnant with her fourth child. She regained her pre-pregnancy weight quickly after delivery and continued to exercise regularly, eat well, and control her body weight after the birth of this child. She has not experienced hyperglycemia since this pregnancy.

Home Medications: Ondansetron and loperamide.

History of Current Illness: After her diagnosis of ovarian cancer, Mona underwent a hysterectomy, bilateral oophorectomy, and salpingectomy; removal of the omentum and surrounding lymph nodes. Mona's oncologist suggested very aggressive treatment. Mona underwent successful rounds of chemotherapy with six rounds of cisplatin followed by radiation therapy before her surgical procedure. After the radiation therapy, Mona started to experience diarrhea; sometimes up to two stools per day. She underwent additional rounds of chemotherapy with carboplatin after her surgical procedure. Her oncologist was pleased that Mona could maintain her body weight during the majority of these treatments. Mona tolerated her postoperative chemotherapy well except for the last two rounds. Mona experienced many adverse gastrointestinal (GI) side effects from the chemotherapy. While Mona's appetite was poor, the GI symptoms caused the most difficulty for Mona. She experienced abdominal pain, nausea and diarrhea; up to eight times per day. The combination of chemotherapy and radiation therapy caused damage to her small intestine and colon. Two days ago, Mona was diagnosed with pelvic radiation disease and her doctor decided to put her on parenteral nutrition before her nutritional status significantly deteriorated. He justified the parenteral feeds as necessary due to Mona's inability to eat without discomfort, her increasing diarrhea, and her recent weight loss. She was to be admitted to the hospital for central line placement and progression to cyclic parenteral nutrition support.

Hospital Day 1 (Admit): Mona was admitted to the general surgical floor after successful central line placement in the outpatient surgical suite. This new central line was to be used exclusively for parenteral nutrition. A nutrition consult was ordered for parenteral feeds to meet all of Mona's nutritional requirements. In the progress notes, the oncologist made it clear that Mona would be allowed to eat, but this po intake and subsequent pain and diarrhea would "make it impossible for Mona to sustain even a fraction of her nutritional needs." Day 1 medications and IV fluids include D5 NS @ 75 mL/hr, morphine sulphate, and diphenoxylate hydrochloride. Nursing noted overall poor po intake; six liquid stools, adequate urine output, and a soft but tender abdomen. Mona's admit weight was 116 pounds.

Table 7.9: Fasting Comprehensive Metabolic Panel, A/G Ratio, Magnesium, Phosphorus, and Osmolality Obtained on Day 1.

Laboratory Values	Normal Ranges or Values	Mona's Laboratory Values	Mona's Value (WNL, High or Low)	Implications or Assessment
Glucose, mg/dL	70–110	143		
Sodium mEq/L	136–145	150		
Potassium, mEq/L	3.5–5.0	4.9		
Chloride, mEq/L	98–106	109		
CO_2, mEq/L	23–30	33		
BUN, mg/dL	10–20	19		
Creatinine, mg/dL	Female: 0.5–1.1	0.9		
Calcium, mg/dL	9.0–10.5	9.7		
Albumin, g/d	3.5–5.0	3.1		
Total protein, g/dL	6.4–8.3	6.8		
Globulin, g/dL	2.3–3.4	2.8		
Albumin/Globulin ratio	>1.0	1.1		
Bilirubin, total, mg/dL	0.3–1.0	0.9		
ALP, U/L	30–120	110		
ALT, U/L	4–36	38		
AST, U/L	0–35	37		
Phosphorus, mg/dL	3.0–4.5	4.4		
Magnesium, mEq/dL	1.3–2.1	1.9		
Osmolality, mOsm/Kg H_2O	285–295	299		

Table 7.10: Selected Values from Fasting CBC and Differential Obtained on Day 1.

Laboratory Values	Normal Ranges or Values	Mona's Values	Mona's Value (WNL, High or Low)	Implications or Assessment
Hemoglobin, g/dL	Female: 12–16	12		
Hematocrit, %	Female: 37–47	37		
WBC, SI units	5–10	4.6		
Neutrophils, %	55–70	57		
Monocytes, %	2–8	2		
Red blood cell count (RBC), SI units	4.7–6.1	4.5		
Mean corpuscular volume (MCV), fL	80–95	82		
Platelet count SI units	150–400	115		

Table 7.11: Selected Additional Fasting Labs and Vital Signs Obtained on Day 1.

Laboratory Values	Normal Ranges or Values	Mona's Values	Mona's Value (WNL, High or Low)	Implications or Assessment
Prealbumin, mg/dL	15–36	13		
Crp, mg/dL	<1.0	24		
HgbA1C, %	<6.0	4.3		
Triglycerides mg/dL	35–135	105		
Transferrin, mg/dL	Female: 250–380	397		
Transferrin receptor assay (TIR) mg/L	Female: 1.9–4.4	4.6		
Ferritin, ng/mL	Female: 10–150	8		
TIBC, mcg/dL	250–460	469		
Temperature, °F	96.4–99.1	98.4		
Blood pressure, mmHg	Systolic <120 Diastolic <80	110/65		
Pulse, beats/minute	60–100	90		
Respirations: breaths/minute	14–20	15		
Pulse oximetry, %	≤95	99		

Hospital Day 2: Mona reported good pain control with her morphine sulphate. She took short walks around the nursing station and would walk downstairs to the healing garden every afternoon and evening. The nutrition consult was completed with recommendations for full parenteral feeds including recommendations for home cyclic feeds. Once the total parental nutrition was hung, Mona's D5NS IV was discontinued. Nursing noted adequate urine output, a soft and tender abdomen, and poor po intake. Four loose stools were noted on the day 2 nursing I/O report. Nursing noted Mona's weight had increased to 120 lbs. since admit. Day 2 medications include morphine sulphate and diphenoxylate hydrochloride.

Hospital Days 3: After receiving approximately thirty-six hours of parenteral feeds, Mona's TPN was held until 8:00 p.m. on the evening of day 3. Cyclic parenteral feeds were started at this time and Mona was scheduled to be discharged three hours after the cyclic parenteral feeds stopped on the morning of day 4. Nursing continued to report adequate urine output, a soft and tender abdomen, poor po intake, and three loose stools. Day 3 medications include morphine sulphate and diphenoxylate hydrochloride.

Hospital Day 4: Mona tolerated the cyclic parenteral feeds well. She continued to take small amounts of po fluids and solids with continued diarrhea after consumption. Her abdominal pain had diminished and she was frequently seen walking around the hospital. She was discharged home on cyclic parenteral feeds. Discharge medications include morphine sulphate and diphenoxylate hydrochloride.

Table 7.12: BMP, Osmolality, Magnesium, and Phosphorus Obtained on Day 2.

Laboratory Values	Normal Ranges or Values	Mona's Values	Mona's Value (WNL, High or Low)	Implications or Assessment
Glucose, mg/dL	70–110	154		
BUN, mg/dL	10–20	14		
Creatinine, mg/dL	Female: 0.5–1.1	0.8		
Sodium, mEq/L	136–145	138		
Chloride, mEq/L	98–106	104		
Potassium. mEq/L	3.5–5.0	3.9		
CO_2, mmol/L	23–30	26		
Osmolality, mOsm/Kg H_2O	285–295	291		
Phosphorus, mg/dL	3.0–4.5	4.1		
Magnesium, mEq/dL	1.3–2.1	1.9		

Case Evaluation

Prioritize Problems and Identify Interprofessional Care

1. List in order of importance Mona's medical/nutritional concerns.

2. Review the concerns listed in question 1. Which member of the health-care team should address each concern and how should the concern be addressed?

Disease Process and Laboratory Interpretation

3. Are there laboratory values or vital signs above that would be a concern regarding Mona's condition upon her admit to the hospital?

4. **a.** What is refeeding syndrome?

   b. What specific labs are altered with refeeding syndrome? How are they altered?

    c. What must one do to with regards to nutrition support to prevent refeeding syndrome in patients at risk?

5. What is your evaluation of the trends in Mona's labs on days 1 and 2 with regards to risk of refeeding syndrome? Do you feel Mona is at risk for developing refeeding syndrome? Explain

6. a. Describe what is potentially happening with Mona's small intestine and colon to prevent her from adequately absorbing nutrients.

    b. Is what you described in question 6a affecting Mona's overall fluid status? Explain.

Anthropometric and Nutrition Assessment

7. a. What is your evaluation of Mona's height/weight status upon admit to the hospital for central line placement and initiation of parenteral feeds?

    b. Describe the significance of Mona's weight gain on hospital day 2. How will this affect her lab values?

8. What is Mona's overall percentage of weight change over the last nine months? Describe any concerns regarding this weight change.

9. Upon admit to the hospital, can Mona be diagnosed with malnutrition based on the ASPEN/AND guidelines? Explain.

10. You are performing a nutrition-focused physical assessment on Mona while she is in the hospital. Describe what you would expect to find in this assessment.

11. What is your general assessment of Mona's dietary intake since her diagnosis of ovarian cancer?

12. Calculate Mona's total energy and protein requirements for her parenteral feedings. Justify your reasoning for method to determine needs.

13. Mona will be allowed to take oral fluids and foods. At present, her oncologist will not count this as a significant source of nutrition. Describe what will need to happen before you will count this intake as a significant source of nutrition.

Medications

14. Prior to admit Mona was taking ondansetron and loperamide. Describe the main function of these medications and possible adverse side effects or drug-nutrient interactions.

15. At one point, Mona was receiving carboplatin. Describe the main function of carboplatin and possible adverse side effects or drug–nutrient interactions.

16. At one point, Mona was receiving cisplatin. Describe the main function of cisplatin and possible adverse side effects or drug–nutrient interactions.

17. Describe the main function of diphenoxylate hydrochloride. Describe possible adverse side effects or drug–nutrient interactions with this medication.

18. Describe the main functions of Percocet and morphine sulphate. Describe possible adverse side effects or drug–nutrient interactions with these medications.

Nutrition Intervention and Recommendations

19. a. What is your initial 2 in 1 parenteral feeding recommendation for Mona on day 2? Refer to energy and protein needs cited in question 12. Provide recommendations by citing total grams of protein and CHO/day; g/kg protein; glucose infusion rate (GIR); TPN goal rate/hr.

    b. Cite IV fat emulsion (IVFE) total volume infused; grams fat/kg and IVFE infusion rate and duration.

    c. Cite total kcal from TPN and IVFE; % protein kcal, % CHO kcal and % fat kcal; total volume infused.

20. **a.** What is your revised cyclic 2 in 1 parenteral feeding recommendation for Mona on day 4? Refer to energy and protein needs cited in question 12. Provide recommendations by citing total grams of protein and CHO/day; g/kg protein; GIR; TPN goal rate/hr (including specific time frame the cycle will run).

    b. Cite IVFE total volume infused; grams fat/kg and IVFE infusion rate and duration.

    c. Cite total kcal from TPN and IVFE; % protein kcal, % CHO kcal and % fat kcal; total volume infused.

21. Cite your nutrition recommendations for Mona once she can fully tolerate oral intake? Specifically, what dietary modifications would you recommend?

Monitoring and Evaluation; Patient Follow-Up

22. **a.** Once Mona is advanced to her cyclic parenteral feeds, how often should her tolerance and response to her parenteral feedings be evaluated?

    b. Explain how you would evaluate tolerance to parenteral feeds and what specific labs would you monitor?

AND Medical Nutrition Therapy (MNT) Guidelines and Documentation for Dietitians

Nutrition Diagnosis Utilizing the PES Statements:

    a. Day 2—Initial consult

    b. When receiving cyclic parenteral feeds as an outpatient

    c. Eventual diet advancement as an outpatient

Nutrition Intervention and Goals Utilizing AND Terminology:

    a. 2—Initial consult

    b. When receiving cyclic parenteral feeds as an outpatient

    c. Eventual diet advancement as an outpatient

Nutrition Monitoring and Evaluation Utilizing AND Terminology:

a. Day 2—Initial consult

b. When receiving cyclic parenteral feeds as am outpatient

c. Eventual diet advancement as an outpatient

REFERENCE LIST

Barber, Jacqueline R., and Gordon S. Sacks. "Parenteral Nutrition Formulations." *ASPEN Adult Nutrition Support Core Curriculum*, edited by Charles M. Mueller, 2nd ed., American Society of Parenteral and Enteral Nutrition, 2012, pp. 245–64.

Charney, Pamela. "The Nutrition Care Process." *Pocket Guide to Nutrition Assessment*, edited by Pamela Charney and Ainsley Malone, 3rd ed., Academy of Nutrition and Dietetics, 2016, pp. 1–14.

Franz, D., et al. "Gastrointestinal Disease." *ASPEN Adult Nutrition Support Core Curriculum*, edited by Charles M. Mueller, 2nd ed., American Society of Parenteral and Enteral Nutrition, 2012, pp. 426–53.

Ireton-Jones, Carol, and Mary Kristofak Russell. "Food and Nutrient Delivery: Nutrition Support." *Krause's Food and the Nutrition Care Process*, edited by Kathleen Mahn and Janice L. Raymond, 14th ed., Elsevier, 2017, pp. 209–26.

Jenson, Gordon L., et al. "Nutrition Screening and Assessment." *ASPEN Adult Nutrition Support Core Curriculum*, edited by Charles M. Mueller, 2nd ed., American Society of Parenteral and Enteral Nutrition, 2012, pp. 155–69.

Kumpf, Vanessa J., and Jane Gervasio. "Complications of Parenteral Nutrition." *ASPEN Adult Nutrition Support Core Curriculum*, edited by Charles M. Mueller, 2nd ed., American Society of Parenteral and Enteral Nutrition, 2012, pp. 284–97.

Langley, G., and S. Tajchman. "Fluids, Electrolytes and Acid-Base Disorders." *ASPEN Adult Nutrition Support Core Curriculum*, edited by Charles M. Mueller, 2nd ed., American Society of Parenteral and Enteral Nutrition, 2012, pp. 98–120.

Malone, Ainsley, and C. Hamilton. "The Academy of Nutrition and Dietetics/The American Society for Parenteral and Enteral Nutrition Consensus Malnutrition Characteristics: Application in Practice." *Nutrition in Clinical Practice*, vol. 28, 2013, pp. 639–50.

Merck Manual Professional Version, http://www.merckmanuals.com/professional/.

Mirtallo, J. M., and M. Patel. "Overview of Parenteral Nutrition." *ASPEN Adult Nutrition Support Core Curriculum*, edited by Charles M. Mueller, 2nd ed., American Society of Parenteral and Enteral Nutrition, 2012, pp. 234–44.

Morris, K. A., and N. Y. Haboubi. "Pelvic Radiation Therapy: Between Delight and Disaster." *World Journal of Gastrointestinal Surgery*, vol. 7, no. 11, 2015, pp. 279–88, doi:10.4240/wjgs.v7.i11.279.

Nelms, M. N. "Diseases of the Lower Gastrointestinal Tract." *Nutrition Therapy and Pathophysiology*, edited by Marcia Nahikian-Nelms, 3rd ed., Wadsworth, Cengage Learning, 2016, pp. 379–435.

—. "Enteral and Parenteral Nutrition Support." *Nutrition Therapy and Pathophysiology*. By Marcia Nahikian-Nelms, 3rd ed., Wadsworth, Cengage Learning, 2016, pp. 88–114.

Nelms, Marcia, and Diane Habash. "Nutrition Assessment: Foundation of the Nutrition Care Process." *Nutrition Therapy and Pathophysiology*, edited by Marcia Nahikian-Nelms, 3rd ed., Wadsworth, Cengage Learning, 2016.

Pagana, Kathleen Deska, and Timothy James Pagana. *Mosby's Manual of Diagnostic and Laboratory Tests*. Mosby/Elsevier, 2014.

Peterson, Sarah J. "Nutrition Focused Physical Assessment." *Pocket Guide to Nutrition Assessment*, edited by Pamela Charney and Ainsley Malone, 3rd ed., Academy of Nutrition and Dietetics, 2016, pp. 76–102.

Van Leeuwen, Anne, and Bladh Mickey Lynn. *Davis's Comprehensive Handbook of Laboratory and Diagnostic Tests with Nursing Implications*. 6th ed., F.A. Davis, 2015.

Case Study: Thyroid Cancer

Case-Specific Learning Objectives

✓ Determine how different stages of disease and treatment can affect nutritional intake and requirements.

✓ Determine appropriate diet therapy for hypothyroidism.

Our Patient: Maureen B. is a fifty-four-year-old female who works part time as a department manager at a local department store. She is 5 feet 6 inches tall and had a stable weight of 165 pounds for the last few years. Maureen and her husband never had children. She lost her husband to lung cancer three years ago and went through a period of depression for a year before meeting a nice fifty-eight-year-old widower at her church. They have been dating for almost two years and recently became engaged.

Medical and Surgical History: Maureen had bilateral hip replacements two years ago; her years as a high school and college cheerleader caused premature hip degeneration. She suffered from typical childhood illnesses. She had her appendix removed when she was a senior in college.

Home Medications: None.

History of Current Illness: Maureen has been receiving annual physical exams. During her last exam, she complained of increased fatigue, neck pain, difficulty swallowing, and an unintentional weight loss of 10 pounds over the last two months. Her physician noted some items of concern regarding Maureen's thyroid gland in her blood work and ran additional tests and a computed tomography (CT) scan of her neck and thyroid. He also diagnosed Maureen with anemia, told her to eat "foods high in iron," and prescribed some supplements. During evaluation of her thyroid, Maureen was upset at the possibility that she had cancer. She remembered the suffering her husband endured for two years before passing away. Her appetite decreased one day and then she would undergo binge eating of sweets and salty fried foods as well as drinking a bottle of wine the next day. Maureen was diagnosed with stage 1 papillary carcinoma of the thyroid gland. The CT scan revealed that there was no involvement of the surrounding lymph nodes. Her physician told Maureen and her fiancée that her prognosis for a full recovery was excellent; however, Maureen remained nervous. The plan of treatment consisted of a tumor biopsy, radiation therapy, and finally a thyroidectomy. She had not lost any additional weight during this work up for thyroid cancer due to her eating and drinking habits.

The outpatient tumor biopsy was uneventful. Maureen underwent three individual rounds of radiation therapy one week apart prior to her thyroidectomy. Maureen did not tolerate the radiation therapy well. She complained of fatigue and nausea lasting two to three days after each radiation treatment. Between the time of the tumor biopsy and the completion of the radiation treatments, Maureen lost an additional 14 pounds.

Table 7.13: Fasting Comprehensive Metabolic Panel Obtained Prior to Initial Doctor's Appointment

Laboratory Values	Normal Ranges or Values	Maureen's Values	Maureen's Value (WNL, High or Low)	Implications or Assessment
Glucose, mg/dL	70–110	123		
Sodium mEq/L	136–145	144		
Potassium, mEq/L	3.5–5.0	4.8		
Chloride, mEq/L	98–106	101		
CO_2, mEq/L	23–30	27		
BUN, mg/dL	10–20	14		
Creatinine, mg/dL	Female: 0.5–1.1	0.8		
Calcium, mg/dL	9.0–10.5	9.0		
Albumin, g/d	3.5–5.0	3.3		
Total protein, g/dL	6.4–8.3	6.5		
Globulin, g/dL	2.3–3.4	2.5		
Bilirubin, total, mg/dL	0.3–1.0	1.0		
ALP, U/L	30–120	100		
ALT, U/L	4–36	30		
AST, U/L	0–35	30		

Table 7.14: Selected Fasting Values from CBC Obtained Prior to Initial Doctor's Appointment.

Laboratory Values	Normal Ranges or Values	Maureen's Values	Maureen's Value (WNL, High or Low)	Specific Implications or Assessment
Hemoglobin, g/dL	Female: 12–16	11		
Hematocrit, %	Female: 37–47	35		
WBC, SI units	5–10	8.2		
Red blood cell count (RBC), SI units	Female: 4.2–5.4	3.6		
Mean corpuscular volume (MCV), fL	80–95	105		
Mean corpuscular hemoglobin (MCH), pg	27–31	35		
Platelet count SI units	150–400	145		

Table 7.15: Selected Additional Fasting Labs and Vital Signs Obtained Prior to Initial Doctor's Appointment.

Laboratory Values	Normal Ranges or Values	Maureen's Values	Maureen's Value (WNL, High or Low)	Implications or Assessment
Prealbumin, mg/dL	15–36	14		
Crp, mg/dL	<1.0	12		
HgbA1C, %	<6.0	5.4		
Transferrin, mg/dL	Female: 250–380	380		
Ferritin, ng/mL	Female: 10–150	134		
TIBC, mcg/dL	250–460	460		
T3, ng/dL	>50: 40–180	165		
Total T4, mcg/dL	Female: 5–12	10		
Free T4, ng/dL	0.8–2.8	2.4		
TBG, mg/dL	1.7–3.6	1.6		
TSH, mU/L	0.3–5	0.8		

Hospital Admit (Day 1): Maureen reported to the outpatient surgical center at the local hospital for a total thyroidectomy. As planned after surgery, Maureen was admitted to the general surgical floor for forty-eight hours of observation before discharge. She was npo for the first twenty-four hours post-op. Day 1 medications include analgesics, SSI (no insulin provided), and synthroid. She received an IV of D5 NS at 85 mL/hr to maintain adequate urine output.

Hospital Days 2 and 3: Maureen felt well other than some neck and incisional pain which was controlled with analgesics. Her incision looked good and the surgeon was pleased with her swallowing so she was offered a clear liquid diet for breakfast on hospital day 2 and advanced to a "diet as tolerated" for subsequent meals. Overall, Maureen ate approximately 40% of each meal as it was painful when she swallowed. Medications include analgesics, SSI (no insulin provided), and synthroid. Maureen's IV fluids of D5 NS was decreased to 40 mL/hr as her po intake of fluids had increased. Urine output remained adequate. She was discharged home before lunch on hospital day 3.

— —

Case Evaluation

Prioritize Problems and Identify Interprofessional Care

1. List in order of importance Maureen's medical/nutritional concerns while she is undergoing radiation therapy.

2. Review the concerns listed in question 1. Which member of the health-care team should address each concern and how should the concern be addressed?

3. List in order of importance Maureen's long term nutritional concerns after her thyroidectomy.

4. Review the concerns listed in question 3. Which member of the health-care team should address each concern and how should the concern be addressed?

Disease Process and Laboratory Interpretation

5. Are there laboratory values or vital signs above that would be a concern regarding Maureen's condition prior to her diagnosis of thyroid cancer?

6. Maureen was diagnosed with "anemia." Specifically, what type of anemia is present and what micronutrients should the doctor have prescribed?

7. Are there laboratory values or vital signs that should be monitored regularly after Maureen's thyroidectomy? Why?

8. After her successful surgery, Maureen will have hypothyroidism. Describe this condition and note any nutrition-related side effects that Maureen may experience.

Anthropometric and Nutrition Assessment

9. What is your evaluation of Maureen's height/weight status prior to her thyroidectomy?

10. Maureen's body weight had dropped from her usual weight of 165 pounds to 141 pounds prior to her thyroidectomy. What percentage of weight loss did Maureen experience and what is the significance of this loss?

11. Upon admit to the hospital, can Maureen be diagnosed with malnutrition based on the ASPEN/AND guidelines? Explain.

12. Assume the RDN performed nutrition focused physical exam on Maureen while she was in the hospital. Describe what you would expect to see from the results of this physical exam.

13. **a.** Calculate Maureen's total energy and protein requirements immediately after her thyroidectomy. Justify your reasoning for method to determine needs.

    b. How would you reassess Maureen's long-term total energy and protein requirements after her thyroidectomy? Justify your reasoning for method to determine needs.

Medications

14. Maureen will require lifelong thyroid hormone replacement. Describe side effects, drug–nutrient interactions, or nutritional concerns with this hormone replacement therapy.

15. Maureen was diagnosed with anemia and prescribed supplements prior to her thyroidectomy. If she develops the same type of anemia in the future will these supplements cause any concern with her synthroid administration?

Nutrition Intervention and Recommendations

16. The diet technician screened Maureen after her admit to the hospital and noted her cancer diagnosis, postoperative status, and recent weight loss. Maureen has been referred to the RDN for consultation. You thoroughly review her medical record and note that Maureen will be discharged from the hospital tomorrow. What suggestions do you have for Maureen regarding her appetite, po intake, and nutritional status for her post-op and long-term nutritional well-being?

Monitoring and Evaluation; Patient Follow-Up

17. Describe a desired nutritional care follow-up schedule for Maureen and what should be addressed at follow-up appointments.

Academy of Nutrition and Dietetics (AND) Medical Nutrition Therapy (MNT) Guidelines and Documentation for Dietitians

Nutrition Diagnosis Utilizing the PES Statements:

a. Hospital day 2

b. As an outpatient on synthroid

Nutrition Intervention and Goals Utilizing AND Terminology:

a. Hospital day 2

b. As an outpatient on synthroid

Nutrition Monitoring and Evaluation Utilizing AND Terminology:

a. Hospital day 2

b. As an outpatient on synthroid

REFERENCE LIST

American Cancer Society, http://www.cancer.org/.

Charney, Pamela. "The Nutrition Care Process." *Pocket Guide to Nutrition Assessment*, edited by Pamela Charney and Ainsley Malone, 3rd ed., Academy of Nutrition and Dietetics, 2016, pp. 1–14.

Cohen, Deoborah A., and Kathryn Sucher. "Neoplastic Disease." *Nutrition Therapy and Pathophysiology*, edited by Marcia Nahikian-Nelms, 3rd ed., Wadsworth, Cengage Learning, 2016, pp. 729–54.

Dean, Sheila. "Medical Nutrition Therapy for Thyroid, Adrenal and Other Endocrine Disorders." *Krause's Food and the Nutrition Care Process*, edited by Kathleen Mahn and Janice L. Raymond, 14th ed., Elsevier, 2017, pp. 619–30.

Hamilton, Kathryn, and Barbara Grant. "Medical Nutrition Therapy for Cancer Prevention, Therapy and Survivorship." *Krause's Food and the Nutrition Care Process*, edited by Kathleen Mahn and Janice L. Raymond, 14th ed., Elsevier, 2017.

Jenson, Gordon L., et al. "Nutrition Screening and Assessment." *ASPEN Adult Nutrition Support Core Curriculum*, edited by Charles M. Mueller, 2nd ed., American Society of Parenteral and Enteral Nutrition, 2012, pp. 155–69.

Malone, Ainsley, and Cynthia Hamilton. "The Academy of Nutrition and Dietetics/The American Society for Parenteral and Enteral Nutrition Consensus Malnutrition Characteristics: Application in Practice." *Nutrition in Clinical Practice*, vol. 28, 2013, pp. 639–50.

Mendelsohn, Robin, and Mark Shattner. "Cancer." *ASPEN Adult Nutrition Support Core Curriculum*, edited by Charles M. Mueller, 2nd ed., American Society of Parenteral and Enteral Nutrition, 2012, pp. 412–25.

Merck Manual Professional Version. http://www.merckmanuals.com/professional/nutritional-disorders/nutrition,-c-,-general-considerations/nutrient-drug-interactions.

—, http://www.merckmanuals.com/professional/.

Nelms, Marcia Nahikian. "Diseases of the Endocrine System." *Nutrition Therapy and Pathophysiology*, edited by Marcia Nahikian-Nelms, 3rd ed., Wadsworth, Cengage Learning, 2016.

Nelms, Marcia, and Diane Habash. "Nutrition Assessment: Foundation of the Nutrition Care Process." *Nutrition Therapy and Pathophysiology*, edited by Marcia Nahikian-Nelms, 3rd ed., Wadsworth, Cengage Learning, 2016.

Pagana, Kathleen Deska, and Timothy James Pagana. *Mosby's Manual of Diagnostic and Laboratory Tests*. Mosby/Elsevier, 2014.

Peterson, Sarah. "Nutrition Focused Physical Assessment." *Pocket Guide to Nutrition Assessment*, edited by Pamela Charney and Ainsley Malone, 3rd ed., Academy of Nutrition and Dietetics, 2016, pp. 76–102.

Van Leeuwen, Anne, and Bladh Mickey Lynn. *Davis's Comprehensive Handbook of Laboratory and Diagnostic Tests with Nursing Implications*. 6th ed., F.A. Davis, 2015.

CHAPTER **8**

Hepatic, Pancreatic and Renal Concerns

- -

Case Study: Hepatic Disease—Part 1: Alcoholic Hepatitis and Ascites

Case-Specific Learning Objectives

- ✓ Determine appropriate diet therapy for stages of hepatic disease.
- ✓ Determine how different stages of disease and treatment can affect nutritional requirements and intake.

Our Patient: Doug V. is a forty-three-year-old Caucasian male who resides in government-assisted housing and receives a monthly disability check due to chronic back pain and emotional distress. He is very good friends with Sarah who lives in the apartment next door and Doug frequently goes to a local bar with her. Sarah is unemployed and receives disability benefits due to bipolar disorder. Doug has held a variety of jobs, primarily janitorial, after graduating from high school. Doug was in special education classes throughout high school due to "emotional issues." Doug received psychological counseling when pursuing his studies in high school, but has refused counseling since turning 18. He has been unemployed for the past seven years after injuring his back at work. He was married at the age of thirty and divorced three years later. He never had children. He started smoking when he was eighteen years old and started drinking when he was sixteen. Doug reports he has never taken illicit drugs, but does "smoke weed" every weekend and has done so since high school. Doug lost his driver's license five years ago and currently relies on the bus to get to doctors' appointments and the grocery store. Every month, Doug also travels to the food bank to pick up a food box and he has a hot meal every day at noon at the community center. The community center is six blocks away from Doug's apartment and he typically walks there with Sarah. Sometimes, they do not make it to the community center and instead stop at a bar on the way.

Medical and Surgical History: Doug experienced typical childhood illnesses. Doug underwent hernia repair eight years ago and notes chronic back pain for the last seven years. "Psychological" issues are briefly noted in Doug's medical history but no definitive diagnosis is noted and Doug denies a history of a psychological diagnosis. Doug has a history of three concussions after falls including two falls off bar stools while intoxicated. He broke his right arm after another fall while intoxicated. He has been hospitalized for alcoholic hepatitis three times over the last two years. Doug was diagnosed with alcoholic hepatitis two years ago. He was diagnosed with a fatty liver and mild ascites nine months ago.

Home Medications: MVI and furosemide.

History of Current Illness: Doug arrived one hour late to his routine three-month check-up. The office receptionist and triage nurse both noticed the smell of alcohol when Doug spoke to them. Doug reported he has been consuming more alcohol over the last ten days to help ease his back pain. Doug reports his waist appears to have grown larger since his last doctor's appointment. Doug cited his appetite has been poor due to his back pain. He also noted that he has not been able to go to the local food bank to pick up his food box, nor has he been able to go to the community center for his regular noon hot meal due to his back pain.

Nutrition focused PE in doctor's office: Upon examination of muscle mass, a slight depression in the temporalis muscle is noted, the acromion process slightly protrudes, and there is a mild depression around the scapula. Upper arm and lower extremity muscle mass appears less developed. Abdominal girth appeared larger than expected based on evaluation of Doug's trunk; however, there is no baseline waist circumference to compare. Current waist circumference measured 38 inches. Grip strength with the hand grip dynamometer was noted to be below average for age. Faint ridging on the fingernails and thin sparse hair was noted. The whites of Doug's eyes had several broken blood vessels and appeared red.

Doug is 5 feet 10 inches tall and currently weighs 67.7 kg. Three months ago, at his doctor's appointment, Doug weighed 65.3 kg.

Table 8.1: Fasting Comprehensive Metabolic Panel, BUN/Creatinine, and A/G Ratios Obtained One Week Prior to Doctors Appointment.

Laboratory Values	Normal Ranges or Values	Doug's Laboratory Values Three Months Ago	Doug's Current Laboratory Values	Doug's Trend (Improving, Stable, Worsening)	Implications or Assessment
Glucose, mg/dL	70–110	90	81		
Sodium mEq/L	136–145	144	136		
Potassium, mEq/L	3.5–5.0	4.2	3.3		
Chloride, mEq/L	98–106	103	100		
CO_2, mEq/L	23–30	24	24		
BUN, mg/dL	10–20	15	12		
Creatinine, mg/dL	Male: 0.6–1.2	0.6	0.6		
BUN/Creatinine ratio	10–20	25	20		
Calcium, mg/dL	9.0–10.5	9.2	9.2		
Albumin, g/d	3.5–5.0	3.4	3.2		
Total protein, g/dL	6.4–8.3	6.4	6.2		
Globulin, g/dL	2.3–3.4	3.4	2.4		
Albumin/ Globulin ratio	>1.0	1.0	1.33		
Bilirubin, total, mg/dL	0.3–1.0	0.8	1.0		
ALP, U/L	30–120	115	125		
ALT, U/L	4–36	34	39		
AST, U/L	0–35	33	42		

Table 8.2: Selected Values from Fasting Complete Blood Count and Differential Obtained One Week Prior to Doctors Appointment.

Laboratory Values	Normal Ranges or Values	Doug's Laboratory Values Three Months Ago	Doug's Current Laboratory Values	Doug's Trend (Improving, Stable, Worsening)	Implications or Assessment
Hemoglobin, g/dL	Male: 14–18	16	14		
Hematocrit, %	Male: 42–52	43	41		
WBC, SI units	5–10	9.5	11.3		
Platelet count SI units	150–400	175	165		

Table 8.3: Selected Additional Labs and Vital Signs Obtained One Week Prior to Doctors Appointment.

Laboratory Values	Normal Ranges or Values	Doug's Laboratory Values Three Months Ago	Doug's Current Laboratory Values	Doug's Trend (Improving, Stable, Worsening)	Implications or Assessment
Crp, mg/dL	<1.0	2.2	4.5		
Ammonia, mcg/dL	10–80	57	76		
INR	0.8–1.1	1.0	0.9		
Alcohol, mg/dL	0	0	0.065		
Magnesium, mEq/L	1.3–2.1	1.4	1.4		
Transferrin, mg/dL	Male: 215–365	385	405		
Ferritin, ng/mL	Male: 12–300	13	10		
Temperature, °F	96.4–99.1	98.2	101.4		
Blood pressure, mmHg	Systolic <120 Diastolic <80	115/80	170/115		
Pulse, beats/ minute	60-100	80	75		
Respirations: breaths/minute	14-20	18	18		
Pulse oximetry, %	≤95	98	98		

— —

Case Evaluation

Prioritize Problems and Identify Interprofessional Care

1. List in order of importance Doug's medical/nutritional concerns.

2. Review the concerns listed in question 1. Which member of the health-care team should address each concern and how should the concern be addressed?

Disease Process and Laboratory Interpretation

3. Are there laboratory values or vital signs above that would be a concern regarding Doug's condition? Explain.

4. Describe your evaluation of the findings from Doug's nutrition focused physical exam.

5. Are there additional blood tests or physical exams you would like to perform to determine if Doug has specific nutrient deficiencies? Explain.

6. Describe three chronic nutritional concerns that may be associated with alcoholic hepatitis or advancing hepatic disease? Describe how these concerns can lead to a diagnosis of malnutrition.

7. **a**. Doug has been diagnosed with a fatty liver and ascites. Describe these conditions.

   b. How can a fatty liver and ascites affect Doug's oral intake and nutritional status?

8. Describe the different Child–Pugh classes of cirrhosis.

Anthropometric and Nutrition Assessment

9. What is your evaluation of Doug's height/weight status at his most recent doctor's appointment?

10. a. What percentage of body weight change has Doug experienced over the past three months?

b. What is the cause or significance of this weight change?

11. At this most recent doctor's appointment, can Doug be diagnosed with malnutrition based on the ASPEN/AND guidelines? Explain.

12. Calculate Doug's total energy and protein requirements. Justify your reasoning for method to determine needs.

13. What is your general assessment of Doug's overall nutritional intake prior to this most recent doctor's appointment?

14. Can you determine if Doug may have a diet deficient in energy, protein, or micronutrients based on his physical exam? Explain.

15. Explain the significance of Doug's recent weight gain.

Medications

16. Why was a MVI prescribed for Doug?

17. Do you feel Doug needs additional micronutrient supplementation? Explain.

18. a. Describe the main function of furosemide. Describe possible adverse side effects or drug–nutrient interactions with this medication.

    b. Review Doug's labs. Are there labs that are depressed due to this medication? Explain.

Nutrition Intervention and Recommendations

19. Based on Doug's medical history and status (weight, labs, etc.), what specific recommendations would you make to increase the energy, protein, and micronutrient content of Doug's diet?

20. Doug currently has been diagnosed with alcoholic hepatitis. Describe dietary modifications for this condition.

21. Assuming Doug develops advancing liver disease. Describe diet modifications for
    a. Cirrhosis

    b. Encephalopathy

Monitoring and Evaluation; Patient Follow-Up

22. Please describe a desired nutritional care follow-up schedule for Doug and what should be addressed at follow-up appointments.

23. What specific dietary questions would you ask Doug in a follow-up to see if he understands his prescribed diet?

24. Do you feel Doug will be compliant with his diet upon discharge? Explain.

Academy of Nutrition and Dietetics (AND) Medical Nutrition Therapy (MNT) Guidelines and Documentation for Dietitians

Nutrition Diagnosis Utilizing the PES Statements:

Nutrition Intervention and Goals Utilizing AND Terminology:

Nutrition Monitoring and Evaluation Utilizing AND Terminology:

REFERENCE LIST

Charney, Pamela. "The Nutrition Care Process." *Pocket Guide to Nutrition Assessment*, edited by Pamela Charney, and Ainsley Malone, 3rd ed., Academy of Nutrition and Dietetics, 2016, pp. 1–14.

Thomas, Frazier, et al. "Liver Disease." *ASPEN Adult Nutrition Support Core Curriculum*, Charles M. Mueller, 2nd ed., American Society of Parenteral and Enteral Nutrition, 2012, pp. 412–25.

Hasse, Jeanetta, and Laura Matarese. "Medical Nutrition Therapy for Hepatobiliary and Pancreatic Disorders." *Krause's Food and the Nutrition Care Process*, edited by Kathleen Mahn, and Janice L. Raymond, 14th ed., Elsevier, 2017.

Jenson, Gordon L., et al. "Nutrition Screening and Assessment." *ASPEN Adult Nutrition Support Core Curriculum*, edited by Charles M. Mueller, 2nd ed., American Society of Parenteral and Enteral Nutrition, 2012, pp. 155–69.

Malone, Ainsley, and Cynthia Hamilton. "The Academy of Nutrition and Dietetics/The American Society for Parenteral and Enteral Nutrition Consensus Malnutrition Characteristics: Application in Practice." *Nutrition in Clinical Practice*, vol. 28, 2013, pp. 639–50.

Merck Manual Professional Version: http://www.merckmanuals.com/professional/nutritional-disorders/nutrition,-c-,-general-considerations/nutrient-drug-interactions.

Nelms, Marcia, and Diane Habash. "Nutrition Assessment: Foundation of the Nutrition Care Process." *Nutrition Therapy and Pathophysiology*, edited by Marcia Nahikian-Nelms, 3rd ed., Wadsworth, Cengage Learning, 2016.

Pagana, Kathleen Deska, and Timothy James Pagana. *Mosby's Manual of Diagnostic and Laboratory Tests*. Mosby/Elsevier, 2014.

Peterson, Sarah J. "Nutrition Focused Physical Assessment." Pocket Guide to Nutrition Assessment, edited by Pamela Charney, and Ainsley Malone, 3rd ed., Academy of Nutrition and Dietetics, 2016, pp. 76–102.

Sucher, Kathryn, and Mattfeldt-Beman Mildred. "Diseases of the Liver, Gallbladder and Exocrine Pancreas." *Nutrition Therapy and Pathophysiology*, edited by Marcia Nahikian-Nelms, 3rd ed., Wadsworth, Cengage Learning, 2016, pp. 436–68.

Van Leeuwen, Anne, and Mickey Lynn Bladh. *Davis's Comprehensive Handbook of Laboratory and Diagnostic Tests with Nursing Implications*, 6th ed., F.A. Davis, 2015.

Case Study: Hepatic Disease—Part 2: Inpatient with Cirrhosis, GI Bleeding, and Delirium Tremens

Case-Specific Learning Objectives

✓ Determine appropriate feeding modality in the presence of altered laboratory values and delirium tremens (DT's).

✓ Calculate appropriate enteral nutrition support therapy in advanced liver disease.

Our Patient, Medical, and Surgical History: Please refer to part 1 of this case to obtain pertinent personal, medical, surgical, dietary, and medication history on Doug. Doug was diagnosed with Cirrhosis, Child–Pugh Class B six months ago.

Home Medications: MVI and furosemide.

History of Current Illness: Doug woke up this morning to some acute abdominal pain. His friend Sarah urged him to go to the emergency room (ER) to have this evaluated. Sarah accompanied Doug to the ER, but they did make a stop at the local bar next to the bus stop before going to the hospital. Doug reported he only had one beer at the bar. He has been consuming a six pack and a couple of shots of whiskey each day to help ease his back pain. Doug noticed dark blood-tinged stools two days ago. Doug reports his waist appears to have grown larger since his last routine doctor's appointment five weeks ago. Doug also notes his appetite has been poor for the last two weeks and refused to elaborate on what he ate. When asked about his daily medication use, Doug reports he "thinks" he takes all his pills each day. He may have run out of one or two medications because he "ran out of money for the month." Doug is planning on getting prescription refills in two days when his monthly disability check arrives.

Emergency Room and Admit (Day 1) Events: Doug appeared to be intoxicated upon arrival to the ER. Sarah essentially dropped Doug off at the triage desk in the ER and left the hospital. Once taken back to a room, Doug immediately requested some food and a beer. He cited the food and beer would make his upset stomach feel better. Doug became upset when the doctor told him that he needed to wait until after his exam to eat. Twenty minutes later, Doug had approximately 300 mL of coffee ground emesis. At this time, a nasogastric tube (NGT) was placed and another 300 mL of coffee ground material was suctioned out of Doug's stomach. Later that afternoon, Doug was admitted to the general medical floor with a diagnosis of gastrointestinal bleeding (GIB), ascites, and cirrhosis. Doug remained npo with the NGT draining to gravity. An IV of D5 ½ NS was started at 65 mL/hr. Day 1 medications included a MVI, 1 mg folate po, 100 mg of thiamine po × 3 days, analgesics, furosemide, sliding-scale insulin (SSI), lactulose, and ranitidine. Doug was measured to be 5 feet 10 inches tall and he weighed 70.1 kg.

Table 8.4: Nonfasting Comprehensive Metabolic Panel BUN/Creatinine and A/G Ratios Obtained in the ER.

Laboratory Values	Normal Ranges or Values	Doug's Nonfasting Laboratory Values: ER	Doug's Value (WNL, High or Low)	Implications or Assessment
Glucose, mg/dL	70–110	141		
Sodium mEq/L	136–145	136		
Potassium, mEq/L	3.5–5.0	3.6		
Chloride, mEq/L	98–106	100		
CO_2, mEq/L	23–30	24		
BUN, mg/dL	10–20	28		
Creatinine, mg/dL	Male: 0.6–1.2	0.6		
BUN/Creatinine ratio	10–20	46.7		
Calcium, mg/dL	9.0–10.5	9.0		
Albumin, g/d	3.5–5.0	3.1		
Total protein, g/dL	6.4–8.3	6.2		
Globulin, g/dL	2.3–3.4	2.4		
Albumin/Globulin ratio	>1.0	1.29		
Bilirubin, total, mg/dL	0.3–1.0	1.1		
ALP, U/L	30–120	175		
ALT, U/L	4–36	50		
AST, U/L	0–35	52		

Table 8.5: Selected Values from Nonfasting Complete Blood Count and Differential Obtained in the ER.

Laboratory Values	Normal Ranges or Values	Doug's Laboratory Values: ER	Doug's Value (WNL, High or Low)	Implications or Assessment
Hemoglobin, g/dL	Male: 14–18	14		
Hematocrit, %	Male: 42–52	40		
WBC, SI units	5–10	11.3		
Platelet count SI units	150–400	165		

Table 8.6: Selected Nonfasting Additional Labs and Vital Signs Obtained in the ER.

Laboratory Values	Normal Ranges or Values	Doug's Laboratory Values: ER	Doug's Value (WNL, High or Low)	Implications or Assessment
Crp, mg/dL	<1.0	4.5		
Ammonia, mcg/dL	10–80	86		
INR	0.8–1.1	0.7		
Alcohol, mg/dL	0	0.065		
Magnesium, mEq/L	1.3–2.1	0.9		
Ferritin, ng/mL	Male: 12–300	10		
Osmolality, mOsm/ Kg H$_2$O	285–295	280		
Temperature, °F	96.4–99.1	101.4		
Blood pressure, mmHg	Systolic <120 Diastolic <80	170/115		
Pulse, beats/minute	60–100	75		
Respirations: breaths/ minute	14–20	18		
Pulse oximetry, %	≤95	98		

Hospital Day 3: Doug had minimal NGT drainage over the prior twenty-four hours and all output appeared clear of blood. During 6:00 a.m. rounds, the physicians discussed removing Doug's NGT and starting a po diet. They also noted abdominal girth had increased 4 inches since admit. Paracentesis to remove ascetic fluid prior to the removal of the NGT was scheduled for later that morning. Successful bedside sedation and removal of 3.75 L of ascetic fluid was achieved at 11:00 a.m. During the procedure, the MD noted that Doug was experiencing some tremors and required additional sedation. Doug also appeared more confused immediately prior to the paracentesis. Day 3 medications included MVI, 1 mg folate po, 100 mg of thiamine, analgesics, furosemide, SSI with 6 units administered, lactulose, and ranitidine. Diazepam was added immediately after the paracentesis as the physicians felt Doug appeared to be going into delirium tremens. At this time, Doug was to remain npo as the doctor felt that it was unsafe to provide him with a diet while he was in DT's. Soft restraints were ordered to be placed on Doug's arms and ankles. The physician decided to place a naso-duodenal feeding tube secured with a nasal bridle and ordered a nutrition consult for nasoduodenal feedings while Doug is in active DT's.

Hospital Days 4–9. Doug remained in DT's from days 4–9. During this time, Sarah would occasionally visit; she appeared intoxicated at every visit and was asked to leave. He was agitated and confused. Cortrak verification of placement of the feeding tube needed to be performed daily. Overall, Doug tolerated his enteral feeds well. Since Doug kept pulling out his IV, he received free water flushes via his feeding tube to meet his free water needs.

He did manage to pull out his Foley catheter once during this time. Urine output remained "adequate" and Doug experienced two to three loose stools each day. Doug's DT's resolved on day 8. He became more alert and cooperative. On day 9, Doug was allowed to take sips of liquids and he did so without difficulty. Days 4–9 medications included MVI, diazepam, analgesics, furosemide, SSI with an average of 8 units per day administered, lactulose, and ranitidine

Table 8.7: Fasting Comprehensive Metabolic Panel, BUN/Creatinine, and A/G Ratios Obtained on Days 3 and 8.

Laboratory Values	Normal Ranges or Values	Doug's Laboratory Values Day 3	Doug's Laboratory Values Day 8	Doug's Trend (Improving, Stable, Worsening)	Implications or Assessment
Glucose, mg/dL	70–110	148	133		
Sodium mEq/L	136–145	140	136		
Potassium, mEq/L	3.5–5.0	4.3	3.7		
Chloride, mEq/L	98–106	103	100		
CO_2, mEq/L	23–30	23	25		
BUN, mg/dL	10–20	22	18		
Creatinine, mg/dL	Male: 0.6–1.2	0.6	0.6		
BUN/Creatinine ratio	10–20	36.6	30		
Calcium, mg/dL	9.0–10.5	9.2	9.3		
Albumin, g/d	3.5–5.0	3.4	3.2		
Total protein, g/dL	6.4–8.3	6.4	6.2		
Globulin, g/dL	2.3–3.4	3.6	2.5		
Albumin/ Globulin ratio	>1.0	0.94	1.28		
Bilirubin, total, mg/dL	0.3–1.0	0.8	1.0		
ALP, U/L	30–120	115	120		
ALT, U/L	4–36	33	33		
AST, U/L	0–35	33	35		

Table 8.8: Selected Values from Fasting Complete Blood Count and Differential Obtained on Days 3 and 8.

Laboratory Values	Normal Ranges or Values	Doug's Laboratory Values Day 3	Doug's Laboratory Values Day 8	Doug's Trend (Improving, Stable, Worsening)	Implications or Assessment
Hemoglobin, g/dL	Male: 14–18	13	14		
Hematocrit, %	Male: 42–52	42	43		
WBC, SI units	5–10	9.5	9.3		
Platelet count SI units	150–400	175	185		

Table 8.9: Selected Nonfasting Additional Labs Obtained on Days 3 and 8.

Laboratory Values	Normal Ranges or Values	Doug's Laboratory Values Day 3	Doug's Laboratory Values Day 8	Doug's Trend (Improving, Stable, Worsening)	Implications or Assessment
Crp, mg/dL	<1.0	4.9	12		
Ammonia, mcg/dL	10–80	95	77		
INR	0.8–1.1	0.7	0.9		
Magnesium, mEq/L	1.3–2.1	1.4	1.6		

Hospital Day 10. Doug was advanced to a full diet for breakfast on day 10. He tolerated solid foods well and ate almost 70% of his meal. The doctor told Doug that if he ate lunch well he would be discharged that afternoon. When lunch arrived, Doug ate 80% of the meal and threw the dessert at the nurse. Doug was angry with his nurse because she did not allow Sarah to visit at lunchtime because Sarah was intoxicated. Doug was discharged later that afternoon. Discharge medications were MVI, furosemide, and low dose lactulose.

Case Evaluation

Prioritize Problems and Identify Interprofessional Care

1. List in order of importance Doug's medical/nutritional concerns from admit date through hospital day 3.

2. Review the concerns listed in question 1. Which member of the health-care team should address each concern and how should the concern be addressed?

3. List in order of importance Doug's medical/nutritional concerns on hospital day 9.

4. Review the concerns listed in question 3. Which member of the health-care team should address each concern and how should the concern be addressed?

Disease Process and Laboratory Interpretation

5. Are there laboratory values or vital signs above that would be a concern regarding Doug's condition? Explain.

6. Describe three chronic nutritional concerns that may be associated with cirrhosis or advancing hepatic disease? Describe how these concerns can lead to a diagnosis of malnutrition.

7. Doug develops delirium tremens. Describe this condition.

8. Doug has been admitted with a diagnosis of GIB, cirrhosis Child–Pugh Class B, and ascites. Describe these conditions.

   a. Describe hepatic encephalopathy

   b. Do you feel Doug has hepatic encephalopathy? Explain.

Anthropometric and Nutrition Assessment

9. a. What is your evaluation of Doug's height/weight status upon his presentation to the ER?

   b. What factors may be present that may affect obtaining an accurate body weight for Doug?

10. Can Doug be diagnosed with malnutrition based on the ASPEN/AND guidelines? Explain.

11. Are there specific nutrient deficiencies that can be diagnosed? Explain.

12. a. Calculate Doug's total energy and protein requirements on day 3. Justify your reasoning for method to determine needs.

b. Would you make any changes to the energy and protein requirements in question 12a when you follow-up with Doug on day 9? Explain

13. What is your general assessment of Doug's overall nutritional intake prior to admit?

Medications

14. Why was a MVI, thiamine, and folate prescribed for Doug?

15. Describe the main function of diazepam. Describe possible adverse side effects or drug–nutrient interactions with this medication.

16. a. Describe the main function of furosemide. Describe possible adverse side effects or drug–nutrient interactions with this medication.

b. This medication appears to be affecting Doug's potassium levels. Is there an alternative medication that can be used to minimize the risk of hypokalemia? Explain.

17. Describe the main function of lactulose. Describe possible adverse side effects or drug–nutrient interactions with this medication.

18. Describe the main function of ranitidine. Describe possible adverse side effects or drug–nutrient interactions with this medication.

Nutrition Intervention and Recommendations

19. What is your initial tube feeding recommendation for Doug on day 3? Refer to energy and protein needs cited in question 12a. Provide recommendations by citing enteral product, goal rate/hr. and daily volume to be infused; total kcal, grams protein, ml free water, %RDI, and grams fiber (if indicated).

20. Describe the Cortrak system for feeding tube placement.

21. Describe a nasal bridle and why this was used for Doug?

22. Cite your nutrition recommendations for Doug once his diet was advanced. What specific diet modifications would you recommend?

23. If Doug must remain on furosemide for an extended period of time, what additional dietary recommendations would you provide Doug upon discharge?

Monitoring and Evaluation; Patient Follow-Up

24. How often should Doug's tolerance and response to his enteral feedings be evaluated? Explain how you would evaluate tolerance to enteral feeds and labs you would suggest obtaining.

25. Please describe a desired nutritional care follow-up schedule for Doug after discharge and specifically what should be addressed at follow-up appointments.

26. What specific dietary questions would you ask Doug in a follow-up to see if he understands his prescribed diet?

27. Do you feel Doug will be compliant with his diet upon discharge? Explain

Academy of Nutrition and Dietetics (AND) Medical Nutrition Therapy (MNT) Guidelines and Documentation for Dietitians

Nutrition Diagnosis Utilizing the PES Statements:

Initial Assessment:

Day 3

Day 9

Nutrition Intervention and Goals Utilizing AND Terminology:

Initial Assessment:

Day 3

Day 9

Nutrition Monitoring and Evaluation Utilizing AND Terminology:

Initial Assessment:

Day 3

Day 9

REFERENCE LIST

Bechtold ML, et al. "Nasal Bridles for Securing Nasoenteric Tubes: A Meta-Analysis." *Nutrition in Clinical Practice: Official Publication of the American Society for Parenteral and Enteral Nutrition*, vol. 29, no. 5, 2014, pp. 667–71.

Charney, Pamela. "The Nutrition Care Process." *Pocket Guide to Nutrition Assessment*, edited by Pamela Charney, and Ainsley Malone, 3rd ed., Academy of Nutrition and Dietetics, 2016, pp. 1–14.

Thomas, Frazier, et al. "Liver Disease." *ASPEN Adult Nutrition Support Core Curriculum*, Charles M. Mueller, 2nd ed., American Society of Parenteral and Enteral Nutrition, 2012, pp. 412–25.

Hasse, Jeanetta, and Laura Matarese. "Medical Nutrition Therapy for Hepatobiliary and Pancreatic Disorders." *Krause's Food and the Nutrition Care Process*, edited by Kathleen Mahn, and Janice L. Raymond, 14th ed., Elsevier, 2017.

Jenson, Gordon L., et al. "Nutrition Screening and Assessment." *ASPEN Adult Nutrition Support Core Curriculum*, edited by Charles M. Mueller, 2nd ed., American Society of Parenteral and Enteral Nutrition, 2012, pp. 155–69.

Malone, Ainsley, and Cynthia Hamilton C. "The Academy of Nutrition and Dietetics/The American Society for Parenteral and Enteral Nutrition Consensus Malnutrition Characteristics: Application in Practice." *Nutrition in Clinical Practice*, vol. 28, 2013, pp. 639–50.

Merck Manual Professional Version: http://www.merckmanuals.com/professional/nutritional-disorders/ nutrition,-c-,-general-considerations/nutrient-drug-interactions.

Nelms, Marcia, and Diane Habash. "Nutrition Assessment: Foundation of the Nutrition Care Process." *Nutrition Therapy and Pathophysiology*, edited by Marcia Nahikian-Nelms, 3rd ed., Wadsworth, Cengage Learning, 2016.

Pagana, Kathleen Deska, and Timothy James Pagana. *Mosby's Manual of Diagnostic and Laboratory Tests*. Mosby/Elsevier, 2014.

Peterson, Sarah J. "Nutrition Focused Physical Assessment." *Pocket Guide to Nutrition Assessment*, edited by Pamela Charney, and Ainsley Malone, 3rd ed., Academy of Nutrition and Dietetics, 2016, pp. 76–102.

Sucher, Kathryn, and Mildred Mattfeldt-Beman. "Diseases of the Liver, Gallbladder and Exocrine Pancreas." *Nutrition Therapy and Pathophysiology*, edited by Marcia Nahikian-Nelms, 3rd ed., Wadsworth, Cengage Learning, 2016, pp. 436–68.

Schuckit, Marc A. "Recognition and Management of Withdrawal Delirium (Delirium Tremens)." *New England Journal of Medicine*, vol. 371, 27 Nov. 2014, pp. 2109–13. doi:10.1056/NEJMra1407298.

Van Leeuwen, Anne, and Mickey Lynn Bladh. *Davis's Comprehensive Handbook of Laboratory and Diagnostic Tests with Nursing Implications*, 6th ed., F.A. Davis, 2015.

Case Study: Gallstone Pancreatitis and Pneumonia

Case-Specific Learning Objectives

- ✓ Evaluate ethnic variations of dietary modifications
- ✓ Calculate nutrition support therapy.
- ✓ Evaluate appropriate modalities of nutrition therapy for pancreatitis.
- ✓ Evaluate appropriate modalities of nutrition therapy after a cholecystectomy.

Our Patient: Michelle M. is a forty-eight-year-old divorced mother of one child. She was born in Russia and immigrated to the United States when she was 13 years old. Michelle loves to cook and share her traditional family meals with her son. They frequently eat fish, meat stews, borscht, potatoes, and cabbage. Michelle likes all foods and loves adding sour cream to nontraditional foods to give them a "Russian flair." Michelle has a "sweet tooth." She must have something sweet after every meal, including breakfast. Michelle loves baked desserts and frequently prepares homemade Russian pastries and sweets. She loves cloudberries and is thrilled when her cousin sends her cloudberry preserves. Michelle will frequently have a shot of vodka to end the evening. Michelle works full time at a local department store and is currently attending school to obtain her realtor's license. She loves to ride her bike and take a variety of exercise classes at the local community center. They recently added a class for lifting weights and Michelle loves this class. Her son is currently a sophomore in college and Michelle is helping to fund his studies. Michelle has managed to keep the small house her son grew up in, but has struggled to pay her bills since her divorce six years ago. Her car recently needed over $1,000 in repairs. Michelle has medical insurance with a high deductible and no dental insurance. She is still making payments on the root canal her son needed four months ago. Michelle is 5 feet 6 inches tall and usually weighs 140 lbs.

Medical and Surgical History: Michelle experienced typical childhood illnesses and she has never broken a bone or needed stitches. Her pregnancy with her son was uneventful and she carried him to term. Michelle was diagnosed with cholelithiasis several years ago. The doctor has advised her to have her gallbladder removed before the stones cause a problem; however, she wants to wait until after she gets her real estate license and collects some sales commissions to have her cholecystectomy.

Home Medications: None.

History of Current Illness: Five days prior to admit, Michelle developed a sore throat and cough. Two days prior to admit, the illness seemed to settle into her chest. Michelle started to experience abdominal pains in the right upper quadrant (RUQ) and chills one day prior to admit. The morning of admit she awoke to a 103° fever, more diffuse abdominal pain that radiated to the back and chest pains with coughing. When her son arrived home from his morning classes, he insisted on taking Michelle to the emergency room (ER).

Emergency Room and Day 1 Events: Michelle was in the ER for five hours. During this time, she underwent an abdominal ultrasound as well as a chest, abdominal, and pelvic computed tomography (CT) scan. Imaging tests revealed gallstones and a large gallstone blocking the pancreatic duct, an inflamed pancreas, and bilateral lower lobe pneumonia. She received a surgical consult before she was admitted with the diagnosis of gallstone pancreatitis and pneumonia. Michelle was scheduled to have a cholecystectomy the next afternoon. Day 1 medications included SSI, IV morphine sulfate for pain management and IV levofloxacin and imipenem. Michelle will be npo until after her surgery and received D5 NS IV running at 80 mL/hr to maintain urine output.

Day 2: Michelle underwent her cholecystectomy at 3:30 p.m. The gallbladder was removed without incident, however postoperatively, the anesthesiologist determined, it was best to keep Michelle intubated due to her post-op pulmonary status and pneumonia. Michelle was admitted intubated and sedated to the surgical ICU at 9:00 p.m. Postoperative medications included SSI (16 units provided), IV morphine sulfate, levofloxacin, and imipenem. She was npo with a D5 ½ NS IV running at 80 mL/hr to maintain adequate urinary output.

Day 3: Michelle remained on the ventilator and was stable overnight. Ventilator management allowed Michelle to remain comfortable. There were no changes in her medications or IV fluid rate. During her morning rounds, the surgeon consulted with the pulmonologist and it was determined that Michelle would remain on the ventilator for several more days while the pneumonia resolved. She was pleased with Michelle's overall abdominal exam. While Michelle had some slight incisional tenderness, she denied diffuse abdominal or radiating pain by shaking her head. The surgeon ordered TPN consisting of 60 g of amino acids, standard electrolytes and 300 g CHO/day to run at a goal rate of 80 mL/hr. Per hospital protocol, parenteral feeds undergo incremental advancement during the first twenty-four hours of therapy with goal rate achieved twenty hours after initiation. The surgeon specifically did not order an intravenous fat emulsion (IVFE) piggyback with the parenteral nutrition order due to "pancreatitis." A nutrition consult was generated with the parenteral nutrition order. The D5 NS IV was ordered to decrease to 25 mL/hr once the TPN was advanced to goal rate.

Table 8.10: Fasting Comprehensive Metabolic Panel, BUN/Creatinine, and A/G Ratios Obtained on Days 1 (Admit) and 3.

Laboratory Values	Normal Ranges or Values	Michelle's Laboratory Values Day 1	Michelle's Laboratory Values Day 3	Michelle's Trend (Improving, Stable, Worsening)	Implications or Assessment
Glucose, mg/dL	70–110	190	152		
Sodium mEq/L	136–145	140	141		
Potassium, mEq/L	3.5–5.0	4.4	4.2		
Chloride, mEq/L	98–106	99	100		
CO_2, mEq/L	23–30	23	25		
BUN, mg/dL	10–20	13	15		
Creatinine, mg/dL	Female: 0.5–1.1	0.7	0.8		
BUN/Creatinine ratio	10–20	18.6	18.8		
Calcium, mg/dL	9.0–10.5	10.1	9.9		
Albumin, g/d	3.5–5.0	3.2	3.0		
Total protein, g/dL	6.4–8.3	6.2	6.0		
Globulin, g/dl	2.3–3.4	3.6	3.7		
Albumin/Globulin ratio	>1.0	0.89	0.81		
Bilirubin, total, mg/dl	0.3–1.0	2.7	1.8		
ALP, U/L	30–120	155	120		
ALT, U/L	4–36	36	32		
AST, U/L	0–35	33	30		

Table 8.11: Selected Values from Fasting Complete Blood Count and Differential Obtained on Days 1 and 3.

Laboratory Values	Normal Ranges or Values	Michelle's Laboratory Values Day 1	Michelle's Laboratory Values Day 3	Michelle's Trend (Improving, Stable, Worsening)	Implications or Assessment
Hemoglobin, g/dL	Female: 12–16	14	14		
Hematocrit, %	Female: 37–47	38	37		
WBC, SI units	5–10	16.5	14.3		
Platelet count SI units	150–400	275	285		

Table 8.12: Selected Additional Labs and Vital Signs Obtained on Days 1 and 3.

Laboratory Value	Normal Ranges or Values	Michelle's Laboratory Values Day 1	Michelle's Laboratory Values Day 3	Michelle's Trend (Improving, Stable, Worsening)	Implications or Assessment
Prealbumin, mg/dL	15–36	12	9		
Crp, mg/dL	<1.0	24	47		
HgbA1C, %	<6.0	5.2			
Bilirubin, mg/dL Direct Indirect	0.1–0.3 0.2–0.8	Direct: 2.1 Indirect: 0.6	Direct: 1.3 Indirect: 0.5		
Ammonia, mcg/dL	10–80	43			
Triglycerides, mg/dL	Female: 35–135	75	105		
Amylase, Somogyi units/dL	60–120	544	327		
Lipase, units/L	0–110	305	258		
Lactic acid, mg/dL	Venous: 5–20	Venous: 7.2			
Phosphorus, mg/dL	3.0–4.5	3.1	3.3		
Magnesium, mEq/L	1.3–2.1	1.4	1.9		
Blood pressure, mmHg	Systolic <120 Diastolic <80	170/115	120/75		

Table 8.12: (*continued*)

Laboratory Value	Normal Ranges or Values	Michelle's Laboratory Values Day 1	Michelle's Laboratory Values Day 3	Michelle's Trend (Improving, Stable, Worsening)	Implications or Assessment
Pulse, beats/minute	60–100	95	85		
Respirations: breaths/minute	14–20	18	18		
Pulse oximetry, %	≤95	90	98		

Hospital Day 4: Michelle remained stable on the ventilator. There were no changes in her medications or IV fluid rate. During her morning rounds, the surgeon reviewed your nutrition consultation and changed Michelle's nutrition support therapy to what you recommended. Michelle continued to have some slight incisional tenderness, she denied diffuse abdominal or radiating pain by shaking her head. Urine output was noted to be adequate.

Hospital Days 5–7: Michelle remained stable on the ventilator and was slowly weaned off the ventilator by hospital day 7. During this time, Michelle continued to tolerate her nutrition support therapy. Urine output remained adequate with the nutrition support therapy and D5 NS at 25 mL/hr. Michelle continued to have some slight incisional tenderness and continued to deny diffuse abdominal or radiating pain. Medications on days 5–7 included SSI (10 units provided daily), IV morphine sulfate, levofloxacin, and imipenem.

Table 8.13: Selected Additional Labs Obtained on Days 6 and 8.

Laboratory Values	Normal Ranges or Values	Michelle's Laboratory Values Day 6	Michelle's Laboratory Values Day 8	Michelle's Trend (Improving, Stable, Worsening)	Implications or Assessment
Amylase, Somogyi units/dL	60–120	165	107		
Lipase, SU/L	0–110	125	86		

Hospital Days 8 and 9: Michelle was transferred to the general surgical floor on day 8 and her diet was advanced. Nutrition support was abruptly discontinued by the surgeon as Michelle wanted to eat and noted that she was hungry during morning rounds. Michelle continued to have some slight incisional tenderness and continued to deny diffuse abdominal or radiating pain. Medications were changed to oral analgesics. All other medications were discontinued. Michelle was eating well, denied pain, and was discharged on over-the-counter analgesics on day 9.

— —

Case Evaluation

Prioritize Problems and Identify Interprofessional Care

1. List in order of importance Michelle's medical/nutritional concerns from admit date through day 3.

2. Review the concerns listed in question 1. Which member of the health-care team should address each concern and how should the concern be addressed?

3. List in order of importance Michelle's medical/nutritional concerns on day 7.

4. Review the concerns listed in question 3. Which member of the health-care team should address each concern and how should the concern be addressed?

Disease Process and Laboratory Interpretation

5. Are there laboratory values or vital signs above that would be a concern regarding Michelle's condition upon admit to the hospital?

6. Describe gallstone pancreatitis.

7. Describe how to interpret the trends in amylase and lipase for Michelle when comparing her admit values in the ER to her labs on days 6 and 8.

8. Why do you feel serum ammonia and lactic acid were obtained upon admit?

Anthropometric and Nutrition Assessment

9. What is your evaluation of Michelle's admit height/weight status?

10. Upon admit to the hospital, can Michelle be diagnosed with malnutrition based on the ASPEN/AND guidelines? Explain.

11. Calculate Michelle's total energy, protein, and fluid requirements. Justify your reasoning for method to determine needs.

Medications

12. Describe the main function of levofloxacin. Describe possible adverse side effects or drug–nutrient interactions with this medication.

13. Describe the main function of imipenem. Describe possible adverse side effects or drug–nutrient interactions with this medication.

14. Describe the main function of morphine sulfate. Describe possible adverse side effects or drug–nutrient interactions with this medication.

Nutrition Intervention and Recommendations

15. a. Do you agree with the surgeon ordering nutrition support on day 3? Explain.

    b. Do you agree with the surgeon's order for fat free parenteral nutrition for Michelle? Justify your reasoning.

16. How many total kcal, grams of CHO and mEq of electrolytes are provided with Michelle's D5 ½ NS IV at 80 mL/hr on day 2?

17. a. What does the TPN ordered by the MD provide? Provide total energy, grams protein, grams CHO, glucose infusion rate (GIR), grams fat (total and per kg); percentage of kcal from CHO, protein, and fat.

    b. Is this parenteral therapy adequate to meet Michelle's needs? Refer to question 11 and explain.

18. You are providing a nutrition therapy assessment for Michelle on day 4. What changes would you recommend to the nutrition support therapy ordered by the MD? Note specific recommendations (therapy, rate, and what this provides). Justify your reasoning for these recommendations.

19. What would your recommendations for long-term nutrition be once Michelle is removed from the ventilator? Cite specific feeds/diet and your recommended advancement schedule.

Monitoring and Evaluation; Patient Follow-Up

20. Regarding both parenteral and enteral nutrition support therapy, how often should Michelle's tolerance and response to her nutrition therapy be evaluated while she is in the hospital? Explain specifically what should be monitored and why.

21. Please describe a desired nutritional care follow-up schedule for Michelle after discharge and specifically what should be addressed at follow-up appointments.

Academy of Nutrition and Dietetics (AND) Medical Nutrition Therapy (MNT) Guidelines and Documentation for Dietitians

Nutrition Diagnosis Utilizing the PES Statements:

Day 3, Initial consult

Day 7, after extubation

Nutrition Intervention and Goals utilizing AND terminology:

Day 3, Initial consult

Day 7, after extubation

Nutrition Monitoring and Evaluation utilizing AND terminology:

Day 3, Initial consult

Day 7, after extubation

REFERENCE LIST

Charney, Pamela. "The Nutrition Care Process." *Pocket Guide to Nutrition Assessment*, edited by Pamela Charney, and Ainsley Malone, 3rd ed., Academy of Nutrition and Dietetics, 2016, pp. 1–14.

Thomas, Frazier, et al. "Liver Disease." *ASPEN Adult Nutrition Support Core Curriculum*, Charles M. Mueller, 2nd ed., American Society of Parenteral and Enteral Nutrition, 2012, pp. 412–25.

Hasse, Jeanetta, and Laura Matarese. "Medical Nutrition Therapy for Hepatobiliary and Pancreatic Disorders." *Krause's Food and the Nutrition Care Process*, edited by Kathleen Mahn, and Janice L. Raymond, 14th ed., Elsevier, 2017.

Jenson, Gordon L., et al. "Nutrition Screening and Assessment." *ASPEN Adult Nutrition Support Core Curriculum*, edited by Charles M. Mueller, 2nd ed., American Society of Parenteral and Enteral Nutrition, 2012, pp. 155–69.

Malone, Anisley, and Cynthia Hamilton. "The Academy of Nutrition and Dietetics/The American Society for Parenteral and Enteral Nutrition Consensus Malnutrition Characteristics: Application in Practice." *Nutrition in Clinical Practice*, vol. 28, 2013, pp. 639–50.

Merck Manual Professional Version: http://www.merckmanuals.com/professional/nutritional-disorders/nutrition,-c-,-general-considerations/nutrient-drug-interactions.

Merck Manual Professional Version: http://www.merckmanuals.com/professional/gastrointestinal-disorders/pancreatitis/acute-pancreatitis.

Nahikian Nelms, Marcia. "Metabolic Stress and the Critically Ill." *Nutrition Therapy and Pathophysiology*, edited by Marcia Nahikian-Nelms, 3rd ed., Wadsworth, Cengage Learning, 2016.

Nelms, Marcia, and Diane Habash. "Nutrition Assessment: Foundation of the Nutrition Care Process." *Nutrition Therapy and Pathophysiology*, edited by Marcia Nahikian-Nelms, 3rd ed., Wadsworth, Cengage Learning, 2016.

Pagana, Kathleen Deska, and Timothy James Pagana. *Mosby's Manual of Diagnostic and Laboratory Tests*. Mosby/Elsevier, 2014.

Peterson, Sarah J. "Nutrition Focused Physical Assessment." *Pocket Guide to Nutrition Assessment*, edited by Pamela Charney, and Ainsley Malone, 3rd ed., Academy of Nutrition and Dietetics, 2016, pp. 76–102.

Sucher, Kathryn, and Mildred Mattfeldt-Beman. "Diseases of the Liver, Gallbladder and Exocrine Pancreas." *Nutrition Therapy and Pathophysiology*, edited by Marcia Nahikian-Nelms, 3rd ed., Wadsworth, Cengage Learning, 2016.

Van Leeuwen, Anne, and Mickey Lynn Bladh. *Davis's Comprehensive Handbook of Laboratory and Diagnostic Tests with Nursing Implications*, 6th ed., F.A. Davis, 2015.

Case Study: Progressive Renal Disease

Case-Specific Learning Objectives

✓ Understand how different stages of renal disease can affect nutritional requirements.

✓ Differentiate between different etiologies associated with the development of renal disease.

✓ Identify foods that require limited intake with chronic kidney disease (CKD).

✓ Evaluate ethnic variations of dietary modifications

Our Patient: Manny P. is a forty-nine-year-old male of Hispanic descent. Both of Manny's parents and his wife's parents were born in Mexico. Manny has four siblings—two sisters and two brothers. Manny is married and has one adult child and two grandchildren. Manny's wife is active and healthy. He keeps active by working in the yard, riding his bike, and swimming. He is motivated to exercise and keeps his weight within normal limits to decrease his risk of developing type 2 diabetes and associated complications. He is employed as a civil engineer and has worked for the same company since graduating from college when he was twenty-five years of age. Ten months ago, his company underwent a round of layoffs and some of Manny's colleagues lost their jobs. These past months have been very stressful. During this time, Manny has gained 15 pounds and has forgone some of his regular exercise. Manny is 5 feet 8 inches tall and now weighs 160 pounds.

Medical and Surgical History: Manny suffered the typical childhood illnesses. He had hernia repair when he was thirty-five years old. The only trauma Manny has endured is a sprained ankle while in high school. Manny's father has type 2 diabetes and hypertension. One sister and two brothers have type 2 diabetes. One of Manny's brothers also has hypertension and had a left below-knee amputation (BKA) due to complications from diabetes. Manny's mother and other sister are both healthy and without chronic medical concerns. Manny was diagnosed with hypertension three years ago.

Home Medications and Newly Prescribed Medications: Captopril, microzide, and erythropoietin (prescribed after the initiation of hemodialysis).

History of Current Illness: Nine months ago, Manny's labs at his routine check-up appeared to be trending toward the development of renal problems. Manny's doctor noted an increase in his typical blood pressure and increased the doses of his antihypertensive medications. Manny was scheduled for follow-up appointments to evaluate his renal function every three months. Manny was referred to a Registered Dietitian Nutritionist to receive information regarding predialysis dietary modifications.

At each subsequent appointment, Manny's glomerular filtration rate continued to decrease. At his last appointment, one week ago, Manny's doctor recommended the placement of an arteriovenous fistula for the initiation of hemodialysis three times per week. He was referred to a Registered Dietitian Nutritionist for additional education regarding the new diet to follow after initiation of hemodialysis therapy. Manny had a temporary catheter for hemodialysis placed in his nephrologist's office. This could be used the fistula for hemodialysis could be placed. The nurse at the nephrologist's office gave Manny a booklet regarding what to expect with hemodialysis treatments including a brief list of foods to avoid. He underwent two rounds of hemodialysis before the fistula for hemodialysis was placed in his left forearm in an outpatient procedure. Manny tolerated this procedure well. Manny had a scheduled appointment with the dialysis Registered Dietitian Nutritionist on the day of his third hemodialysis treatment.

Typical Dietary Intake: Manny loves all foods. Manny and his wife typically cook using traditional family recipes three to four days per week. They eat a variety of foods the rest of the week. Manny loves his beans and eggs for breakfast every morning. He goes out to lunch one day each workweek. Manny and his wife also love going to a movie and quick dinner every Friday night. Lately, he has been having two cartons of frozen Greek yogurt for dessert each evening. Manny prefers to drink water and will drink several glasses each day. He prefers coffee with breakfast, iced tea with lunch, and a beer every time he goes out to eat. He will have a margarita with dinner once per week as well. When Manny meets with the RDN to discuss his renal diet he notes that over the last twenty-four hours he ate everything YOU ate or drank.

Table 8.14: Fasting Comprehensive Metabolic Panel, BUN/Creatinine, A/G Ratios, and Osmolality Obtained One Week Prior to Doctor's Appointment Before Initiation of Hemodialysis

Laboratory Values	Normal Ranges or Values	Manny's Laboratory Values	Manny's Value (WNL, High or Low)	Implications or Assessment
Glucose, mg/dL	70–110	123		
Sodium mEq/L	136–145	151		
Potassium, mEq/L	3.5–5.0	5.8		
Chloride, mEq/L	98–106	101		
CO_2, mEq/L	23–30	27		
BUN, mg/dL	10–20	64		
Creatinine, mg/dL	Male: 0.6–1.2	2.8		
BUN/Creatinine ratio	10:1–20:1	12.9		
Calcium, mg/dL	9.0–10.5	10.2		
Albumin, g/d	3.5–5.0	3.2		
Total protein, g/dL	6.4–8.3	6.2		
Globulin, g/dL	2.3–3.4	2.3		
Albumin/Globulin ratio	>1.0	1.39		
Bilirubin, total, mg/dL	0.3–1.0	1.0		
ALP, U/L	30–120	87		
ALT, U/L	4–36	15		
AST, U/L	0–35	23		

Table 8.15: Selected Additional Fasting Labs and Vital Signs Obtained One Week Prior to Doctor's Appointment Before Initiation of Hemodialysis

Laboratory Values	Normal Ranges or Values	Manny's Laboratory Values	Manny's Value (WNL, High or Low)	Implications or Assessment
Prealbumin, mg/dL	15–36	39		
Crp, mg/dL	<1.0	14		
HgbA1C, %	<6.0	6.0		
Transferrin, mg/dL	215–365 (M)	388		
TIBC, mcg/dL	250–460	472		
Phosphorus, mg/dL	3.0–4.5	5.2		
Magnesium, mEq/dL	1.3–2.1	2.3		
Creatinine clearance, mL/min	Male: 85–125 Decrease 6–7 mL/min for each decade over 40	52		
GFR, mL/mn/1.73 m2	<15 for dialysis	14		
Temperature, °F	96.4–99.1	98.4		
Blood pressure, mmHg	Systolic <120 Diastolic <80	170/115		
Pulse, beats/ minute	60–100	75		
Respirations: breaths/minute	14–20	18		
Pulse oximetry, %	≤95	98		

Case Evaluation

Prioritize Problems and Identify Interprofessional Care

1. List in order of importance Manny's medical/nutritional concerns nine months prior to the development of CKD.

2. Review the concerns listed in question 1. Which member of the health-care team should address each concern and how should the concern be addressed?

3. List in order of importance Manny's medical/nutritional concerns once Manny was diagnosed with CKD and starting hemodialysis treatments.

4. Review the concerns listed in question 3. Which member of the health-care team should address each concern and how should the concern be addressed?

Disease Process and Laboratory Interpretation

5. Describe the progression of renal disease through the four different stages leading up to CKD (stage 5) requiring either hemodialysis or peritoneal dialysis. Include expected laboratory and physiologic changes with each stage.

6. **a.** There are several risk factors associated with the development of CKD. Describe risk factors that can increase one's risk of developing CKD and specifically how these risk factors affect renal function.

   b. What risk factors for CKD where present in Manny's medical history?

7. Describe the differences between peritoneal dialysis and hemodialysis.

8. Prior to the initiation of hemodialysis, are there laboratory values above that would be a concern regarding Manny's renal status?

9. **a.** Can you determine if Manny has anemia based on the labs above? If so, what type of anemia does Manny have and why is this present?

   b. Describe Manny's risk of developing anemia in the future and include why he is at risk.

    c. Assuming Manny develops anemia and continues to struggle with anemia. Describe how would this be reflected in a nutrition focused physical exam?

Anthropometric and Nutrition Assessment:

10. What is your evaluation of Manny's current height/weight status?

11. Prior to the initiation of hemodialysis, can Manny be diagnosed with malnutrition based on the ASPEN/AND guidelines? Explain.

12. **a.** Why would you expect to see changes in Manny's weight from the time-frame immediately before to immediately after hemodialysis?

    b. If Manny gains too much weight between dialysis treatments what specific nutrition related concerns would you address with Manny?

13. Calculate Manny's total energy and protein requirements. Justify your reasoning for method to determine needs.

Medications

14. Describe the main function of captopril. Describe possible adverse side effects or drug–nutrient interactions with this medication.

15. Describe the main function of microzide. Describe possible adverse side effects or drug–nutrient interactions with this medication.

16. Describe the main functions of erythropoietin. Describe possible adverse side effects or drug–nutrient interactions with this medication.

17. Describe recommended micronutrient supplementation for hemodialysis patients and why these supplements are recommended.

18. a. Medications and their metabolites may be excreted by the kidneys. Describe precautions that must be considered with medications administered to patients with CKD in the predialysis phase.

b. Medications and their metabolites may be excreted by the kidneys. Describe precautions that must be considered with medications administered to patients with CKD who receive scheduled hemodialysis or peritoneal dialysis.

Nutrition Intervention and Recommendations

19. Assume you saw Manny nine months prior to the diagnosis of CKD. Describe specific diet recommendations would you make regarding Manny's diet?

20. Manny has been diagnosed with CKD. Describe specific diet recommendations would you make regarding Manny's diet?

21. Describe additional nutritional/dietary requirements, restrictions, or supplementation that may be required if Manny did not have CKD, but instead developed nephrolithiasis.

22. Describe the progression of dietary modifications including energy and protein needs through the four different stages of kidney disease leading up to CKD and subsequent hemodialysis or peritoneal dialysis.

23. Describe the National Renal Diet. Would this be appropriate for Manny? Explain.

Monitoring and Evaluation; Patient Follow-Up

24. Please describe the recommended nutritional care follow-up schedule for CKD patients undergoing hemodialysis.

25. What specific dietary questions would you ask Manny in follow-up appointments to see if he understands his prescribed diet?

26. Manny had bloodwork obtained after one month of three times weekly hemodialysis treatments. These fasting labs were obtained prior to Manny's hemodialysis treatment. Based on the labs in Table 8.16, what specific nutritional concerns should be addressed at Manny's follow-up appointment with the RDN?

Table 8.16: Selected Fasting Comprehensive Metabolic Panel, Osmolality, and Additional Labs Obtained Predialysis after One Month of Hemodialysis Treatments.

Laboratory Values	Normal Ranges	Manny's Fasting Laboratory Values	Manny's Value (WNL, High or Low)	Implications or Assessment	Expected Change in Labs After Hemodialysis
Glucose, mg/L	70–110	148			
BUN, mg/dL	10–20	72			
Creatinine, mg/dL	0.6–1.2	2.7			
Sodium, mEq/L	136–145	151			
Chloride, mEq/L	98–106	110			
Potassium. mEq/L	3.5–5.0	6.2			
CO_2, mmol/L	23–30	29			
Osmolality, mOsm/Kg H_2O	285–295	312			
pH	7.35–7.45	7.31			

(Continued)

Table 8.16: (*continued*)

Laboratory Values	Normal Ranges	Manny's Fasting Laboratory Values	Manny's Value (WNL, High or Low)	Implications or Assessment	Expected Change in Labs After Hemodialysis
Phosphorus, mg/dL	3.0–4.5	5.8			
Magnesium, mEq/dL	1.3–2.1	2.6			
Albumin, g/d	3.5–5.0	3.3			
Prealbumin, mg/dL	15–36	30			
Crp, mg/dL	<1.0	4			
Hemoglobin, g/dL	Male: 14–16	14			
Hematocrit, %	Male: 42–52	39			
Red blood cell count (RBC), SI units	4.7–6.1	4.9			
Mean corpuscular volume (MCV), fL	80–95	83			
Transferrin, mg/dL	Male: 215–365	344			
TIBC, mcg/dL	250–460	432			

Academy of Nutrition and Dietetics (AND) Medical Nutrition Therapy (MNT) Guidelines and Documentation for Dietitians.

Nutrition Diagnosis Utilizing the PES Statements:

Predialysis

At initiation of hemodialysis

After one month of hemodialysis treatments

Nutrition Intervention and Goals Utilizing AND Terminology:

Predialysis

At initiation of hemodialysis

After one month of hemodialysis treatments

Nutrition Monitoring and Evaluation Utilizing AND Terminology:

Predialysis

At initiation of hemodialysis

After one month of hemodialysis treatments

REFERENCE LIST

Charney, Pamela. "The Nutrition Care Process. " *Pocket Guide to Nutrition Assessment*, edited by Pamela Charney, and Ainsley Malone, 3rd ed., Academy of Nutrition and Dietetics, 2016, pp. 1–14.

Collier, Scott, and Michael J. Landram. "Treatment of Prehypertension: Lifestyle and/or Medication." *Vascular Health Risk Management*, vol. 8, 2012, pp. 613–19.

Malone, Ainsley, and Cynthia Hamilton. "The Academy of Nutrition and Dietetics/The American Society for Parenteral and Enteral Nutrition Consensus Malnutrition Characteristics: Application in Practice." *Nutrition in Clinical Practice*, vol. 28, 2013, pp. 639–50.

Merck Manual Professional Version, http://www.merckmanuals.com/professional/nutritional-disorders/nutrition,-c-,-general-considerations/nutrient-drug-interactions.

National Kidney Foundation. https://www.kidney.org/.

National Kidney Foundation Kidney Disease Outcomes Quality Initiative. https://www.kidney.org/professionals/guidelines.

Nelms, Marcia, and Diane Habash. "Nutrition Assessment: Foundation of the Nutrition Care Process." *Nutrition Therapy and Pathophysiology*, edited by Marcia Nahikian-Nelms, 3rd ed., Wadsworth, Cengage Learning, 2016.

Nahikian Nelms, Marcia. "Metabolic Stress and the Critically Ill." *Nutrition Therapy and Pathophysiology*, edited by Marcia Nahikian-Nelms, 3rd ed., Wadsworth, Cengage Learning, 2016.

Pagana, Kathleen Deska, and Timothy James Pagana. *Mosby's Manual of Diagnostic and Laboratory Tests*. St. Louis, MO: Mosby/Elsevier, 2014.

Peterson, Sarah J. "Nutrition Focused Physical Assessment." *Pocket Guide to Nutrition Assessment*, edited by Pamela Charney, and Ainsley Malone, 3rd ed., Academy of Nutrition and Dietetics, 2016, pp. 76–102.

van Leeuwen, Anne, and Mickey Lynn Bladh. *Davis's Comprehensive Handbook of Laboratory and Diagnostic Tests with Nursing Implications*, 6th ed., F.A. Davis, 2015.

Wilkens, Katy J., et al. "Medical Nutrition Therapy for Renal Disorders." Krause's Food and the Nutrition Care Process, edited by Kathleen Mahn, and Janice L. Raymond, 14th ed., Elsevier, 2017, pp. 700–28.

Wolk, Robert, and Charles I. Fouks. "Renal Disease." *ASPEN Adult Nutrition Support Core Curriculum*, Charles M. Mueller, 2nd ed., American Society of Parenteral and Enteral Nutrition, 2012, pp. 491–510.

CHAPTER 9

Respiratory Concerns

- -

Case Study: Chronic Obstructive Pulmonary Disease Exacerbation and Respiratory Failure

Case-Specific Learning Objectives

- ✓ Assess physical data from a nutrition-focused physical exam.
- ✓ Plan enteral nutrition support therapy.
- ✓ Plan transitional feedings advancing to oral intake.
- ✓ Plan calorie and nutrient dense nutrition therapy.

Our Patient: Jack K. is a sixty-seven-year-old retired fireman. Jack is married, and has two children and five grandchildren. He started smoking when he was twenty-one years old and quit seventeen years ago after suffering a burn and inhalational injury at work. Jack and his wife who is a retired nurse love to travel. They go on at least one big vacation and several small vacations each year. They would spend a month on the east coast each summer visiting their son and three of their grandchildren. Jack's daughter, her husband and their two children live a mile from Jack and his wife. Jack's daughter has been helping her mom more over the last year since Jack fell off his bike and broke his wrist and ankle. Jack's wife feels that Jack has slowed down since this bike accident, but Jack refuses to admit this has happened. Jack did not want to take an annual big trip this year, which is the first time this has happened since his retirement at age sixty.

Medical and Surgical History: Jack experienced typical childhood illnesses. He was active in high school and college sports and suffered ankle and knee sprains in various team sports. Jack suffered a 12% burn to his bilateral upper extremities and inhalation injury when he was working a large fire seventeen years ago. This injury prompted Jack to quit smoking; however, he was diagnosed with chronic obstructive pulmonary disease (COPD) after this event. Jack required surgical repair of both his right wrist and right ankle after falling off his bike a year ago. He was in physical therapy for six months after these procedures.

Home Medications: Jack has theophylline and albuterol inhalers. He takes roflumilast once per day.

History of Current Illness: Jack's COPD flared up during his surgery to repair his broken wrist and ankle one year ago. The expected two-day hospital stay was lengthened to a week. Jack was in the progressive care unit needing frequent breathing treatments from the respiratory therapist to maintain proper lung function. After this hospitalization, Jack's medication doses to treat his COPD were increased. While in physical therapy, the twice-weekly sessions would wear Jack out. He needed a nap after each session. Jack did regain good range of motion with his injured wrist and ankle, but Jack was happy to have his physical therapy sessions end as they were "exhausting." Over the past year, Jack's wife noted that his appetite decreased and he lost weight. She had to buy him new clothes due to the weight loss. During this time, Jack would take more naps and was less active. Jack appeared to struggle more with breathing during any activity. Over the last month, Jack would have difficulty breathing when taking a shower, doing minor yard work, or when playing with his school-aged grandchildren. Jack and his wife both became concerned when his grandchildren developed a sore throat and cold prior to the Thanksgiving holiday. Jack's wife always cooked a big Thanksgiving dinner for the entire family. His son, daughter in law, and grandchildren who live on the east coast always come home for Thanksgiving. Jack had five coughing grandchildren in his home Thanksgiving weekend. Jack was so tired that he lounged on the sofa for most of the holiday weekend. His appetite was poor, his throat was sore, and he was having difficulty berating. Jack woke up early in the morning the Monday after Thanksgiving. He told his wife he was having difficulty breathing and needed to go to the emergency room (ER). She was worried about his weight loss and wanted him to eat before they left for the hospital; he refused.

Emergency Room and Day 1 Events: By the time, Jack and his wife arrived at the local ER, Jack was in acute respiratory distress and complained of pain when breathing. His pain was noted to be a 6 out of 10 on the pain scale. He was sedated and nasally intubated. His wife told the ER physician that Jack is 6 feet tall. She noted that he weighed 160 pounds at his doctors' appointment one month ago. Jack remained in the ER for several hours and once he was stabilized, he was transferred to the Medical Intensive Care Unit (MICU) where he would remain on the ventilator. His diagnosis upon admit to the MICU included COPD exacerbation, acute respiratory distress syndrome (ARDS) and pneumonia. Upon arrival to the MICU, the RN weighed Jack and he weighed 72.5 kg. IV fluids consisting of D5NS at 40 mL/hr, a 500-mL bolus of lactated ringer's solution, and 25 g of a 5% IV albumin solution were ordered. These solutions assisted in normalizing fluid and electrolyte status. During the first day of his ICU stay, Jack was able to maintain adequate urine output. The physician noted that she expected Jack to remain intubated for several days and ordered feeding tube placement and a nutrition consult. Day 1 medications include levofloxacin, *furosemide,* analgesics, sedatives, theophylline, sliding-scale insulin (ssi), and prednisone.

Table 9.1: Fasting Basic Metabolic Panel and Osmolality Obtained in ER.

Laboratory Values	Normal Ranges or Values	Jack's Laboratory Values: Pre-Op	Jack's Value (WNL, High or Low)	Implications or Assessment
Glucose, mg/dL	70–110	135		
BUN, mg/dL	10–20	12		
Creatinine, mg/dL	Male: 0.6–1.2	0.5		
Sodium, mEq/L	136–145	131		
Chloride, mEq/L	98–106	96		
Potassium, mEq/L	3.5–5.0	3.2		
CO_2, mmol/L	23–30	31		
Osmolality, mOsm/kg H_2O	285–295	281		

Table 9.2: Selected Fasting Additional Labs and Vital Signs Obtained in the ER.

Laboratory Values	Normal Ranges or Values	Jack's Laboratory Values: Pre-Op	Jack's Value (WNL, High or Low)	Implications or Assessment
Prealbumin, mg/dL	15–36	12		
CRP, mg/dL	<1.0	20		
Albumin, g/dL	3.5–5.0	2.5		
HgbA1C, %	<6.0	5.2		
Phosphorus, mg/dL	3.0–4.5	2.7		
Magnesium, mEq/dL	1.3–2.1	1.3		
Temperature, °F	96.4–99.1	103.1		
Blood pressure, mmHg	Systolic <120 Diastolic <80	165/105		
Pulse, beats/minute	60–100	100		
Respirations, breaths/minute	14–20	30		
Pulse oximetry, %	≤95	86		

Table 9.3: Selected Fasting Values from Complete Blood Count and Differential Obtained in ER.

Laboratory Values	Normal Ranges or Values	Jack's Laboratory Values:	Jack's Value (WNL, High or Low)	Implications or Assessment
Hemoglobin, g/dL	Male: 14–18	12		
Hematocrit, %	Male: 42–52	41		
WBC, SI units	5–10	14.2		
Lymphocytes, %	20–40	48		
Neutrophils, %	55–70	95		
Platelet count SI units	150–400	315		

Table 9.4: Jack's ABG's Upon Admit to the ICU on Mechanical Ventilation.

Laboratory Values	Normal Ranges or Values	Jack's Laboratory Values: ICU	Jack's Value (WNL, High or Low)	Implications or Assessment
pH	7.35–7.45	7.35		
PCO_2, mmHg	35–45	48		
HCO_3, mEq/L	21–28	27		
PO_2, mmHg	80–100	82		
O_2 sat, %	95–100	96		
Base excess, mEq/L	0 ± 2	−1		

Hospital Day 2: Jack remained intubated, sedated, and was resting comfortably. He denied pain. The IV of D5NS was increased to 60 mL/hr and nursing reported adequate urine output. The Registered Dietitian Nutritionist (RDN) performed a nutrition-focused physical exam on Jack. Enteral feeding goals were provided as well. Day 2 medications include levofloxacin, furosemide analgesics, sedatives, theophylline, ssi (5 units administered), and prednisone.

Nutrition-Focused Physical Exam Completed by the RDN: Pitting edema, 3+ in the bilateral lower extremities and 2+ edema in the bilateral upper extremities was noted. Mucous membranes and eyes appeared moist. Fingernails appeared to be of normal shape and appearance except for poor blanching. A slight depression in the temporalis muscle and a slight protrusion of the acromion bone were noted with difficulty to assess additional muscles due to edema.

Table 9.5: Basic Metabolic Panel and Osmolality Obtained on Day 2.

Laboratory Values	Normal Ranges or Values	Jack's Laboratory Values: Pre-Op	Jack's Value (WNL, High or Low)	Implications or Assessment
Glucose,mg/dL	70–110	154		
BUN, mg/dL	10–20	15		
Creatinine, mg/dL	Male: 0.6–1.2	0.7		
Sodium, mEq/L	136–145	141		
Chloride, mEq/L	98–106	99		
Potassium, mEq/L	3.5–5.0	3.9		
CO_2, mmol/L	23–30	28		
Osmolality, mOsm/kg H_2O	285–295	289		

Table 9.6: Selected Additional Labs Obtained on Day 2.

Laboratory Values	Normal Ranges or Values	Jack's Laboratory Values: Pre-Op	Jack's Value (WNL, High or Low)	Implications or Assessment
Phosphorus, mg/dL	3.0–4.5	2.7		
Magnesium, mEq/dL	1.3–2.1	1.3		

Table 9.7: Selected Values from Complete Blood Count and Differential Obtained on Day 2.

Laboratory Values	Normal Ranges or Values	Jack's Laboratory Values	Jack's Value (WNL, High or Low)	Implications or Assessment
Hemoglobin, g/dL	Male: 14–18	13		
Hematocrit, %	Male: 42–52	43		
WBC, SI units	5–10	11.7		
Lymphocytes, %	20–40	40		
Neutrophils, %	55–70	75		
Platelet count SI units	150–400	320		

Table 9.8: Jack's ABG's on Mechanical Ventilation on Day 3.

Laboratory Values	Normal Ranges or Values	Jack's Laboratory Values: ICU	Jack's Value (WNL, High or Low)	Implications or Assessment
pH	7.35–7.45	7.39		
PCO_2, mmHg	35–45	41		
HCO_3, mEq/L	21–28	25		
PO_2, mmHg	80–100	89		
O_2 sat, %	95–100	98		
Base excess, mEq/L	0 ± 2	0		

Hospital Days 3–7. Jack remained intubated, sedated, and was resting comfortably. He continued to deny pain with breathing, however, he did not like the endotracheal (ET) tube in his throat. The tube feeding recommended by the RDN was advanced to goal rate on day 3 and nursing reported Jack tolerated this advancement. During this time, Jack's abdomen remained soft and nontender, he had a soft bowel movement (BM) daily and adequate urine output was noted. The IV of D5NS remained at 40 mL/hr. Days 3–7 medications include levofloxacin, furosemide analgesics, sedatives, theophylline, and ssi (an average of 6–10 units per day was administered). The prednisone dose was started to be weaned down on day 5 with plans to discontinue by day 8.

Hospital Days 8–9. Jack continued to respond to treatment and was weaned from the ventilator just after midnight on day 8. He received albuterol breathing treatments several times during the day and tolerated them well. He was able to start taking po liquids at breakfast. He tolerated them well and the physician ordered removal of the feeding tube and advancement of the diet. He was transferred to the general medical floor at 7:00 p.m. that night. Jack ate 40% of each meal, continued with his albuterol treatments and walked around the medical floor after being transferred. Jack continued to improve and was discharged home at 1:00 p.m. on day 9.

Case Evaluation

Prioritize Problems and Identify Interprofessional Care

1. List in order of importance Jack's medical/nutritional concerns from admit through day 2.

2. Review the concerns listed in question 1. Which member of the healthcare team should address each concern and how should the concern be addressed?

3. List in order of importance Jack's medical/nutritional concerns at discharge.

4. Review the concerns listed in question 3. Which member of the healthcare team should address each concern and how should the concern be addressed?

Disease Process and Laboratory Interpretation

5. Upon admit, are there laboratory values or vital signs that would be a concern regarding Jack's condition? Explain.

6. Review the trends in Jack's ABG's by comparing Tables 9.4 and 9.8. What is your overall assessment of the trend/changes in these labs?

7. Describe two to three chronic nutritional concerns that may be associated with COPD? Describe how these concerns can lead to a diagnosis of malnutrition.

8. What do the labs tell us about Jack's fluid status in the ER?

Anthropometric and Nutrition Assessment

9. a. What is your evaluation of Jack's height/weight status upon admit to the ER? Are there factors present that may affect obtaining an accurate body weight for Jack?

b. What is your assessment of Jack's body weight at his doctor's appointment one month prior to his admit to the hospital?

10. Can Jack be diagnosed with malnutrition based on the ASPEN/AND guidelines? Explain.

11. Can you determine if Jack may have had a preadmit diet deficient in energy, protein, or micronutrients based on his nutrition focused physical exam? Explain.

12. Calculate Jack's total energy and protein requirements. Justify your reasoning for method to determine needs.

Medications

13. Jack took roflumilast once per day prior to his admit. Describe the main function of roflumilast, possible adverse side effects or drug–nutrient interactions with this medication.

14. Describe the main function of levofloxacin. Describe possible adverse side effects or drug–nutrient interactions with this medication.

15. Describe the main function of theophylline. Describe possible adverse side effects or drug–nutrient interactions with this medication.

16. Describe the main function of furosemide. Describe possible adverse side effects or drug–nutrient interactions with this medication.

17. Describe the main function of prednisone. Describe possible adverse side effects or drug–nutrient interactions with these medications.

18. Describe why an albumin IV was given to Jack?

Nutrition Intervention and Recommendations

19. The physician ordered placement of a feeding tube. What type of tube would you recommend for Jack (NG, nasoduodenal, PEG, etc.) and why?

20. What is your tube feeding recommendation for Jack? Refer to energy and protein needs cited in question 12. Provide recommendations by citing enteral product, goal rate/hr, and daily volume to be infused; total kcal, grams protein, ml free water, %RDI, and grams fiber, (if indicated).

21. On day 8, the physician recommended stopping Jack's tube feeding and starting a diet. Do you agree with this or would you recommend a nutritional therapy transition? Describe.

22. Cite your nutrition recommendations for Jack once his diet was advanced. Specifically, what diet would you recommend and why?

Monitoring and Evaluation; Patient Follow-Up

23. How often should Jack's tolerance and response to his enteral feedings be evaluated? Explain how you would evaluate tolerance to enteral feeds and labs you would suggest obtaining.

24. Please describe a desired out-patient nutrition care follow-up schedule for Jack and specifically what should be addressed at follow-up appointments.

Academy of Nutrition and Dietetics (AND) Medical Nutrition Therapy (MNT) Guidelines and Documentation for Dietitians

Nutrition Diagnosis Utilizing the PES Statements:

Initial consult:

Once diet advanced:

Nutrition Intervention and Goals Utilizing AND Terminology:

Initial consult:

Once diet advanced:

Nutrition Monitoring and Evaluation Utilizing AND Terminology:

Initial consult:

Once diet advanced:

REFERENCE LIST

American Lung Association. http://www.lung.org/.

Ayers, Phil, et al. "Acid-Base Disorders: Learning the Basics." *Nutrition in Clinical Practice*, vol. 30, 2015, pp. 14–20.

Bergman, Ethan, and Susan Hawk. "Diseases of the Respiratory System." *Nutrition Therapy and Pathophysiology*, edited by Marcia Nahikian-Nelms, 3rd ed., Wadsworth, Cengage Learning, 2016.

Charney, Pamela. "The Nutrition Care Process." *Pocket Guide to Nutrition Assessment*, edited by Pamela Charney and Ainsley Malone, 3rd ed., Academy of Nutrition and Dietetics, 2016, pp. 1–14.

Jenson, Gordon L., et al. "Nutrition Screening and Assessment." *ASPEN Adult Nutrition Support Core Curriculum*, edited by Charles M. Mueller, 2nd ed., American Society of Parenteral and Enteral Nutrition, 2012, pp. 155–69.

Langley, Ginger, and Sharla Tajchman. "Fluids, Electrolytes and Acid-Base Disorders." *ASPEN Adult Nutrition Support Core Curriculum,* edited by Charles M. Mueller, 2nd ed., American Society of Parenteral and Enteral Nutrition, 2012, pp. 98–120.

Malone, Ainsley, and Cynthia Hamilton. "The Academy of Nutrition and Dietetics/The American Society for Parenteral and Enteral Nutrition Consensus Malnutrition Characteristics: Application in Practice." *Nutrition in Clinical Practice*, vol. 28, 2013, pp. 639–50.

Merck Manual Professional Version. http://www.merckmanuals.com/professional/nutritional-disorders/nutrition,-c-,-general-considerations/nutrient-drug-interactions.

Mueller, Donna H. "Medical Nutrition Therapy for Pulmonary Disease." *Krause's Food and the Nutrition Care Process*, edited by Kathleen Mahn and Janice L. Raymond, 14th ed., Elsevier, 2017, pp. 782–98.

Nelms, Marcia, and Diane Habash. "Nutrition Assessment: Foundation of the Nutrition Care Process." *Nutrition Therapy and Pathophysiology*, edited by Marcia Nahikian-Nelms, 3rd ed., Wadsworth, Cengage Learning, 2016.

Pagana, Kathleen Deska, and Timothy James Pagana. *Mosby's Manual of Diagnostic and Laboratory Tests*. Mosby/Elsevier, 2014.

Peterson, Sarah J. "Nutrition Focused Physical Assessment." *Pocket Guide to Nutrition Assessment*, edited by Pamela Charney and Ainsley Malone, 3rd ed., Academy of Nutrition and Dietetics, 2016, pp. 76–102.

Turner, Krista. "Pulmonary Failure." *ASPEN Adult Nutrition Support Core Curriculum*, edited by Charles M. Mueller, 2nd ed., American Society of Parenteral and Enteral Nutrition, 2012, pp. 412–25.

Van Leeuwen, Anne, and Mickey Lynn Bladh. *Davis's Comprehensive Handbook of Laboratory & Diagnostic Tests with Nursing Implications*, 6th ed., F. A. Davis, 2015.

— —

Case Study: Inpatient with History of Chronic Obstructive Pulmonary Disease and Cholecystitis Requiring Surgery and Mechanical Ventilation

Case-Specific Learning Objectives

- ✓ Assess physical data from a nutrition-focused physical exam.
- ✓ Evaluate clinical and laboratory factors to assess acid–base balance.
- ✓ Plan enteral nutrition support therapy.
- ✓ Plan transitional feedings advancing to oral intake.

Our Patient: Mary H. is a sixty-eight-year-old retired dental hygienist. She is married, has two children and four grandchildren. She smoked for twenty-five years before quitting at age forty-five. Since retiring Mary has been very active with her husband. They love to travel and would typically go to National Parks to hike each summer. Due to Mary's respiratory status, the trips have become less adventuresome the last five years. Mary has been taking yoga classes two or three evenings per week for the last two years.

Medical and Surgical History: As a child, Mary suffered from the typical childhood illnesses. She had a tonsillectomy at age six and an appendectomy at age ten. She delivered both children via C-section greater than thirty-five years ago. Mary was diagnosed with chronic obstructive pulmonary disease (COPD) five years ago and osteopenia four years ago. Mary started to experience right upper quadrant (RUQ) pain after eating a little over a year ago and was diagnosed with cholelithiasis. At that time, Mary switched to a lower fat diet to alleviate adverse symptoms associated with her gallbladder. Two months ago, her doctor advised Mary to have her gallbladder electively removed. Mary wanted to wait until after her sister came to visit to have this elective procedure and scheduled an elective laparoscopic cholecystectomy for the week following her sister's visit.

Home Medications: Mary routinely uses a theophylline inhaler, and takes calcium with vitamin D supplements twice daily. She takes naproxen sodium two to three times per week for general "pains." Mary takes alendronate once per week.

History of Current Illness: Two weeks ago, Mary's sister and her husband arrived for a visit from the Midwest. Mary and her sister cooked a lot of their favorite meals from childhood. The two couples ate their evening meals in restaurants every other night. Mary commented that she had been eating a "spicier and higher fat" diet since the arrival of her sister. The couples would enjoy a bottle of wine with snacks of nuts, cheese and crackers, veggies and dips, or fruit before dinner each evening. Mary noted for the week prior to admit that her abdominal pain had been worsening after meals. Two days prior to admit, Mary complained of dyspnea, nausea, and abdominal pain; especially after meals. She had been unable to eat for twenty-four hours prior to admit. At this time Mary's husband called the doctor and he was advised to take Mary to the local ER for a direct admit and cholecystectomy later in the day.

Admitting Data

Height: 5 feet 4 inches; weight: 120 pounds. Mary reported a usual weight of 110 pounds at her last doctor's appointment and noted the weight gain is probably due to the change in eating habits since the arrival of her sister. She stated she feels "bloated."

Hand grip strength: Below average for age

Selected data from Body Composition analysis with Tanita obtained at doctor's office at last check-up—Body fat percentage: 13.5%

Fat mass: 14.2 pounds; body water percentage: 65%; body water mass: 68.25 pounds.

Fat free mass: 95.8 pounds

Diet: npo

Nutrition-Focused Physical Exam: Nurse documented pitting edema, 2+ in bilateral upper and lower extremities; general pallor; nails with transverse ridging, clubbing, and koilonychias; eyes with pale conjunctiva.

The nurse reports Mary is in mild distress with pain reported as a 7 out of 10.

Hospital Admit (Day 1): Mary was scheduled for a 2:00 p.m. cholecystectomy with plans for discharge that evening. During surgery, Mary developed some breathing difficulties and was unable to be removed from the ventilator. Post-op, she was transferred and admitted to the ICU on a ventilator. IV fluids of D5 ½ NS at 70 mL/hr were ordered to keep her in fluid and electrolyte balance. Mary was to remain npo overnight and her NGT was to remain at low wall suction. Day 1 medications include amoxicillin, analgesics, theophylline, ssi, and prednisone.

Table 9.9: Fasting Basic Metabolic Panel and Osmolality Obtained Pre-Op.

Laboratory Values	Normal Ranges or Values	Mary's Laboratory Values: Pre-Op	Mary's Value (WNL, High or Low)	Implications or Assessment
BUN, mg/dL	10–20	11		
Creatinine, mg/dL	Female: 0.5–1.1	0.7		
Sodium, mEq/L	136–145	136		
Chloride, mEq/L	98–106	97		
Potassium, mEq/L	3.5–5.0	4.0		
CO_2, mmol/L	23–30	31		
Osmolality, mOsm/ kg H_2O	285–295	300		

Table 9.10: Selected Additional Fasting Labs and Vital Signs Obtained Pre-Op.

Laboratory Values	Normal Ranges or Values	Mary's Laboratory Values: Pre-Op	Mary's Value (WNL, High or Low)	Implications or Assessment
Prealbumin, mg/dL	15–36	14		
CRP, mg/dL	<1.0	20		
Albumin, g/dL	3.5–5.0	3.0		
HgbA1C, %	<6.0	5.2		
Bilirubin, total, mg/dL	0.3–1.0	0.7		
Amylase, Somogyi units/dL	60–120	105		
Lipase, units/L	0–110	85		
Lactic acid, mg/dL	Venous: 5–20	5.4 (venous)		
Transferrin receptor assay, mg/L	Female: 1.9–4.4	5.3		
Transferrin, mg/dL	Female: 250–380	395		
Ferritin, ng/mL	Female: 10–150	8		
TIBC, mcg/dL	250–460	475		
Phosphorus, mg/dL	3.0–4.5	3.2		
Magnesium, mEq/dL	1.3–2.1	1.4		
Temperature, °F	96.4–99.1	103.1		
Blood pressure. mmHg	Systolic <120 Diastolic <80	160/110		
Pulse, beats/minute	60–100	100		
Respirations, breaths/minute	14–20	24		
Pulse oximetry, %	≤95	90		

Table 9.11: Selected Values from Fasting Complete Blood Count and Differential Obtained Pre-Op.

Laboratory Values	Normal Ranges or Values	Mary's Laboratory Values: Pre-Op	Mary's Value (WNL, High or Low)	Implications or Assessment
Hemoglobin, g/dL	Female: 12–16	10		
Hematocrit, %	37–47	35		
WBC, SI units	5–10	14.2		
Neutrophils, %	55–70	95		
Platelet count SI units	150–400	315		

Table 9.12: ABG's Upon Admit to the ICU.

Laboratory Values	Normal Ranges or Values	Mary's Laboratory Values: ICU	Mary's Value (WNL, High or Low)	Implications or Assessment
pH	7.35–7.45	7.33		
PCO_2, mmHg	35–45	48		
HCO_3, mEq/L	21–28	24		
PO_2, mmHg	80–100	82		
O_2 sat, %	95–100	96		
Base excess, mEq/L	0 ± 2	–2		

Hospital Day 3: After remaining in stable condition on day 2, the doctor determined that Mary would remain on the ventilator for several more days, so a nasoduodenal feeding tube was placed by the RDN. The MD ordered a nutrition consult for enteral feeding goals. Mary complained of slight abdominal incisional pain. Day 3 medications included amoxicillin, analgesics, theophylline, prednisone, and sliding scale insulin (ssi) (12 units over the last twenty-four hours). D5W was running at 65 mL/hr to maintain adequate urine output.

Hospital Day 5: Mary continued to respond well to the ventilator and current medication therapy. Day 5 medications remained the same as day 3 medications. Her incision appeared to be healing and she complained of minimal incisional or abdominal discomfort. Mary produced a normal bowel movement daily. She continued to receive D5 ½ NS IV at 65 mL/hr to maintain adequate urinary output. She tolerated the enteral feedings that had been recommended with the initial nutrition consult on day 3.

Around noon the surgical resident came by to see Mary. He was concerned with Mary's low albumin level and frail appearance so he decided to increase the tube feeding rate previously recommended by 25 mL/hr.

Table 9.13: Comprehensive Metabolic Panel Day 5 Prior to TF Increase.

Laboratory Value	Normal Ranges or Values	Mary's Laboratory Values: Day 5	Mary's Value (WNL, High or Low)	Implications or Assessment
Glucose, mg/dL	70–110	144		
Sodium, mEq/L	136–145	144		
Potassium, mEq/L	3.5–5.0	4.6		
Chloride, mEq/L	98–106	102		
CO_2, mEq/L	23–30	32		
BUN, mg/dL	10–20	14		
Creatinine, mg/dL	Female: 0.5–1.1	0.8		
BUN/creatinine ratio	10–20	11.2		
Calcium, mg/dL	9.0–10.5	8.7		
Magnesium, mEq/L	1.3–2.1	1.6		
Albumin, g/dL	3.5–5.0	2.3		
Total protein, g/dL	6.4–8.3	5.5		
Globulin, g/dL	2.3–3.4	2.6		
Albumin/globulin ratio	>1.0	0.88		
Bilirubin, total, mg/dL	0.3–1.0	0.7		
ALP, U/L	30–120	100		
ALT, U/L	4–36	27		
AST, U/L	0–35	31		

Table 9.14: ABG's on Hospital Day 5 Prior to TF Increase.

Laboratory Values	Normal Ranges or Values	Mary's Laboratory Values: Day 5	Mary's Value (WNL, High or Low)	Implications or Assessment
pH	7.35–7.45	7.38		
PCO_2, mmHg	35–45	44		
HCO_3, mEq/L	21–28	28		
PO_2, mmHg	80–100	92		
O_2 sat, %	95–100	98		
Base excess, mEq/L	0 ± 2	−0.2		

Hospital Day 6: During your morning rounds checking all your ICU tube fed patients, you noted the surgical resident's change in Mary's tube feeding rate and her most recent ABG's. You reassessed this change in enteral support and made new tube feeding recommendations. Day 6 medications included amoxicillin, analgesics, theophylline, prednisone, and ssi (24 units over the last twenty-four hours). D5W is now running at 45 mL/hr and urine output was noted to be adequate.

Table 9.15: ABG's Day 6.

Laboratory Values	Normal Ranges or Values	Mary's Laboratory Values: Day 6	Mary's Value (WNL, High or Low)	Implications or Assessment
pH	7.35–7.45	7.31		
PCO_2, mmHg	35–45	52		
HCO_3, mEq/L	21–28	27		
PO_2, mmHg	80–100	86		
O_2 sat, %	95–100	98		
Base excess, mEq/L	0 ± 2	−3		

Hospital Days 7–14: Mary continued to progress once enteral feedings were corrected on day 6. She was successfully weaned from the ventilator on day 10. Mary continued to receive theophylline. All other medications and IVs were discontinued by day 10. Enteral feedings continued at goal rate after extubation from the ventilator. Mary started to safely take sips and chips after extubation, but remained on enteral feedings for one more day. It was determined that Mary could advance to a regular consistency diet on day 11 and the surgical resident ordered the removal of the feeding tube. By day 12, she was consistently consuming 35% of her prescribed diet. Mary was discharged from the hospital on day 14.

— —

Case Evaluation

Prioritize Problems and Identify Interprofessional Care

1. List in order of importance Mary's medical/nutritional concerns from admit date through hospital day 3.

2. Review the concerns listed in question 1. Which member of the healthcare team should address each concern and how should the concern be addressed?

3. List in order of importance Mary's medical/nutritional concerns on hospital day 6.

4. Review the concerns listed in question 3. Which member of the healthcare team should address each concern and how should the concern be addressed?

5. List in order of importance Mary's medical/nutritional concerns on hospital days 11 and 12.

6. Review the concerns listed in question 5. Which member of the healthcare team should address each concern and how should the concern be addressed?

Disease Process and Laboratory Interpretation

7. Are there laboratory values or vital signs above that would be a concern regarding Mary's condition upon presentation to the ER?

8. Describe two to three chronic nutritional concerns that may be associated with COPD? Describe how these concerns can lead to a diagnosis of malnutrition.

9. What is your interpretation of Mary's ABG's and acid–base status based on the data in Table 9.12 upon Mary's admit to the ICU?

10. a. Review Mary's ABG's and acid–base status based on the data in Table 9.15 on day 6. What is Mary's acid–base disorder and what is the cause of this acid–base disorder?

    b. Describe additional data in Mary's case to support this conclusion?

Anthropometric and Nutrition Assessment

11. What is your evaluation of Mary's admit height/weight status?

12. What is your overall interpretation of the body composition/physical assessment data? Do these data point to any nutritional concerns? Explain.

13. Would you encourage Mary to gain weight during this hospital stay? Explain.

14. Upon admit, can Mary be diagnosed with malnutrition based on the ASPEN/AND guidelines? Explain.

15. What is your general assessment of Mary's cited nutritional intake prior to her surgery? Was her diet prior to surgery lower or higher in total fat?

16. Can you determine if Mary may have a diet deficient in energy, protein, or micronutrients based on her nutrition-focused physical exam? Explain.

17. Calculate Mary's total energy and protein requirements for your initial assessment on hospital day 3. Justify your reasoning for method to determine needs.

18. How would you reassess Mary's total energy, protein, and overall dietary requirements on hospital day 12 prior to discharge from the hospital. Anticipate Mary's posthospitalization needs when making this follow-up.

Medications

19. Describe the main function of theophylline. Describe possible adverse side effects or drug–nutrient interactions with this medication.

20. Describe the main function of prednisone. Describe possible adverse side effects or drug–nutrient interactions with this medication.

21. Describe the main function of alendronate. Describe possible adverse side effects or drug-nutrient interactions with this medication.

Nutrition Intervention and Recommendations

22. Based on Mary's history and her status upon admit (weight, labs), do you feel it was important for the MD to order enteral feedings immediately post-op or was it appropriate to wait until it was determined if Mary would remain on the ventilator for several days? Explain.

23. Make a recommendation for Mary's goal enteral feedings on day 3. Provide recommendations by citing enteral product, goal rate/hr, and daily volume to be infused; total kcal, grams protein, ml free water, %RDI, and grams fiber provided (if indicated).

24. On day 5, the surgical resident increased Mary's tube feeding recommended in question 23 to a rate that was 25 mL/hr higher than what you recommended. Based on your evaluation of Mary's laboratory data in Table 9.15 on day 6 and your answer to question 10 do you agree with this change? Explain how you would address this issue with the surgical resident. Describe tube feeding changes you would make and why.

25. Once Mary is extubated, what is the appropriate diet that she should receive? Consider her hospital course as well as her medical history when making this decision.

26. Assuming Mary is taking 35% of her prescribed diet twenty-four hours after extubation. Describe how you would like to transition Mary off enteral nutrition support to a full diet.

Monitoring and Evaluation; Patient Follow-Up

27. How often should Mary's tolerance and response to her enteral feedings be evaluated? Explain specifically how you would evaluate tolerance to enteral feeds and labs you would suggest obtaining.

28. Please describe a desired nutritional care follow-up schedule and what should be addressed at follow-up appointments.

29. What specific dietary questions would you ask Mary in a follow-up appointment after discharge to see if she understands her prescribed diet?

Academy of Nutrition and Dietetics (AND) Medical Nutrition Therapy (MNT) Guidelines and Documentation for Dietitians

Nutrition Diagnosis Utilizing the PES statements:

A. Day 3

B. Day 6

C. Day 12

Nutrition Intervention and Goals Utilizing AND Terminology:

    A. Day 3

    B. Day 6

    C. Day 12

Nutrition Monitoring and Evaluation Utilizing AND Terminology:

    A. Day 3

    B. Day 6

    C. Day 12

REFERENCE LIST

American Lung Association. http://www.lung.org/.

Ayers, Phil, et al. "Acid-Base Disorders: Learning the Basics." *Nutrition in Clinical Practice*, vol. 30, 2015, pp. 14–20.

Bergman, Ethan, and Susan Hawk. "Diseases of the Respiratory System." *Nutrition Therapy and Pathophysiology*, edited by Marcia Nahikian-Nelms, 3rd ed., Wadsworth, Cengage Learning, 2016.

Charney, Pamela. "The Nutrition Care Process." *Pocket Guide to Nutrition Assessment*, edited by Pamela Charney and Ainsley Malone, 3rd ed., Academy of Nutrition and Dietetics, 2016, pp. 1–14.

Jenson, Gordon L., et al. "Nutrition Screening and Assessment." *ASPEN Adult Nutrition Support Core Curriculum*, edited by Charles M. Mueller, 2nd ed., American Society of Parenteral and Enteral Nutrition, 2012, pp. 155–69.

Langley, Ginger, and Sharla Tajchman. "Fluids, Electrolytes and Acid-Base Disorders." *ASPEN Adult Nutrition Support Core Curriculum,* edited by Charles M. Mueller, 2nd ed., American Society of Parenteral and Enteral Nutrition, 2012, pp. 98–120.

Malone, Ainsley, and Cynthia Hamilton. "The Academy of Nutrition and Dietetics/The American Society for Parenteral and Enteral Nutrition Consensus Malnutrition Characteristics: Application in Practice." *Nutrition in Clinical Practice*, vol. 28, 2013, pp. 639–50.

Merck Manual Professional Version. http://www.merckmanuals.com/professional/nutritional-disorders/nutrition,-c-,-general-considerations/nutrient-drug-interactions.

Mueller, Donna H. "Medical Nutrition Therapy for Pulmonary Disease." *Krause's Food and the Nutrition Care Process*, edited by Kathleen Mahn and Janice L. Raymond, 14th ed., Elsevier, 2017, pp. 782–98.

Nelms, Marcia, and Diane Habash. "Nutrition Assessment: Foundation of the Nutrition Care Process." *Nutrition Therapy and Pathophysiology*, edited by Marcia Nahikian-Nelms, 3rd ed., Wadsworth, Cengage Learning, 2016.

Pagana, Kathleen Deska, and Timothy James Pagana. *Mosby's Manual of Diagnostic and Laboratory Tests.* Mosby/Elsevier, 2014.

Peterson, Sarah J. "Nutrition Focused Physical Assessment." *Pocket Guide to Nutrition Assessment*, edited by Pamela Charney, and Ainsley Malone, 3rd ed., Academy of Nutrition and Dietetics, 2016, pp. 76–102.

Tanita Professional Products. http://www.tanita.com/es/bc-418/.

Turner, Krista. "Pulmonary Failure." *ASPEN Adult Nutrition Support Core Curriculum*, edited by Charles M. Mueller, 2nd ed., American Society of Parenteral and Enteral Nutrition, 2012, pp. 412–25.

Van Leeuwen, Anne, and Mickey Lynn Bladh. *Davis's Comprehensive Handbook of Laboratory & Diagnostic Tests with Nursing Implications*, 6th ed., F. A. Davis, 2015.

CHAPTER 10

Trauma, Burns, and Wound Care Concerns

- -

Case Study: Burns

Case-Specific Learning Objectives

- ✓ Determine how different stages of injury, treatment, and recovery can affect nutritional requirements and intake.
- ✓ Develop and calculate enteral nutrition support therapy.
- ✓ Interpret results of indirect calorimetry measurements.
- ✓ Understand how medications can affect feeding tolerance.
- ✓ Assess the unique nutritional requirements of a patient with thermal injuries.
- ✓ Calculate Parkland fluid resuscitation needs.
- ✓ Identify and calculate differences between acute care and rehabilitative nutritional requirements.

Our Patient: Craig P. is a twenty-five-year-old male who is employed at a local fast food restaurant. Neighbors report that the rental house Craig shares with his girlfriend appeared to have many visitors arriving, daily, sometimes at odd hours late in the evening. Neighbors have witnessed Craig and his visitors exchanging envelopes or small packages outside the house in the evenings. There are rumors in the neighborhood that Craig works in the "recreational pharmaceutical industry."

Medical and Surgical History: Unremarkable. Craig suffered the typical childhood illnesses. No prior surgical history reported.

Home Medications: None reported.

Emergency Room and Admit (Day 1): At 1:30 a.m., Craig was in a house fire and suffered a 48% total body surface area (TBSA) burn to his BUE, BLE, face, neck, chest, and back. Craig's ankles and feet were not burned as he was wearing socks and shoes at the time of the explosion. The burns on Craig's RLE were circumferential and pulses in the right foot and ankle were diminished. He reported that his girlfriend, who was also injured in the fire, was cooking when the gas stove exploded. Due to the burn occurring in an enclosed space, the presence of facial burns and Craig complaining of hoarseness and dyspnea he was placed on mechanical ventilation at the fire scene and was transported to the local burn center. The firefighters noted that the fire started in the kitchen and based on the appearance at the fire scene there appeared to be supplies indicating crystal methamphetamine was being produced. Firefighters also reported the house appeared to be filthy with dirty plates and containers of rotting food scattered throughout the house. The fire department determined the fire was caused when Craig's methamphetamine lab exploded. Prior to intubation and transport to the local burn center, Craig told the Emergency Medical Technicians (EMTs) he was 5 feet 9 inches tall and weighed 143 pounds.

Upon arrival Craig was placed on the Parkland fluid resuscitation protocol and provided with Parkland fluids in the form of D5W, lactated ringer's, and 25% albumin. A Foley catheter was placed to monitor urine output. Nursing reported adequate hourly urine output achieved during Parkland resuscitation protocol. Craig arrived with soot on his face and singed facial hair. A bronchoscopy and oral exam was performed and the presence of a grade 3 inhalational injury was confirmed by the presence of copious carbonaceous sputum and severe inflammation in the trachea and lungs. It was also noted in the oral exam that Craig's teeth appeared to be in rather poor condition. Wounds were evaluated and all were determined to be third degree. A naso-duodenal feeding tube was placed in the emergency room (ER). After stabilization in the ER, Craig was taken directly to the operating room (OR) for burn wound escharotomies. A four-compartment fasciotomy of the RLE was performed to protect circulation of the right foot. Post-op, Craig was admitted to his intensive care unit (ICU) room intubated, sedated, and in critical condition. Standard post-op orders included a nutrition consult and a standard high-protein enteral formula to start at 50 mL/hr advancing to a goal of 100 mL/hr until the nutrition consult providing revised tube feeding goals is completed. Day 1 medications included wound healing micronutrient supplementation, morphine sulphate, fentanyl, lorazepam, a low dose of dopamine, sliding-scale insulin (SSI); antibiotics including gentamicin, amikacin, and cefazolin; nebulized albuterol, heparin, and mucomyst. Dressing changes using an antimicrobial ointment were ordered BID.

Table 10.1: Nonfasting Comprehensive Metabolic Panel, Osmolality, and Albumin to Globulin (A/G) Ratios Obtained in the ER.

Laboratory Value	Normal Ranges or Values	Craig's Nonfasting Laboratory Values in ER	Craig's Value (WNL, High or Low)	Implications or Assessment
Glucose, mg/dL	70–110	188		
Sodium, mEq/L	136–145	144		
Potassium, mEq/L	3.5–5.0	3.8		
Chloride, mEq/L	98–106	102		
CO_2, mEq/L	23–30	38		
BUN, mg/dL	10–20	22		
Creatinine, mg/dL	Male: 0.6–1.2	1.1		
Calcium, mg/dL	9.0–10.5	8.8		
Albumin, g/dL	3.5–5.0	2.4		
Total protein, g/dL	6.4–8.3	5.7		
Globulin, g/dL	2.3–3.4	3.0		
A/G ratio	>1.0	0.8		
Bilirubin, total, mg/dL	0.3–1.0	1.3		
ALP, U/L	30–120	125		
ALT, U/L	4–36	42		
AST, U/L	0–35	43		
Osmolality, mOsm/kg H_2O	285–295	297		

Table 10.2: Selected Values from Nonfasting Complete Blood Count and Differential Obtained in the ER.

Laboratory Value	Normal Ranges or Values	Craig's Nonfasting Laboratory Values in ER	Craig's Value (WNL, High or Low)	Implications or Assessment
Hemoglobin, g/dL	Male: 14–18	15		
Hematocrit, %	Male: 42–52	42		
WBC, SI units	5–10	16.3		
Platelet count SI units	150–400	298		

Table 10.3: Selected Nonfasting Additional Labs and Vital Signs Obtained in the ER.

Laboratory Value	Normal Ranges or Values	Craig's Nonfasting Laboratory Values in ER	Craig's Value (WNL, High or Low)	Implications or Assessment
Prealbumin, mg/dL	15–36	9		
CRP, mg/dL	<1.0	37		
HgbA1C, %	<6.0	5.4		
Lactic acid, mg/dL	Venous: 5–20	21		
Ammonia, mcg/dL	10–80	38		
INR	0.8–1.1	0.9		
Phosphorus, mg/dL	3.0–4.5	2.1		
Magnesium, mEq/dL	1.3–2.1	1.0		
Alcohol, %	0	0.21		
Cannabis, ng/mL	0	27		
Amphetamines, ng/mL	0	215		
Temperature, °F	96.4–99.1	100.4		
Blood pressure, mmHg	Systolic <120 Diastolic <80	180/105		
Pulse, beats/ minute	60–100	80		
Pulse oximetry, %	≤95	70		

Table 10.4: ABG's Obtained in the ER.

Lab Values	Normal Range	Craig's Laboratory Values in ER	Craig's Value (WNL, High or Low)	Implications or Assessment
pH	7.35–7.45	7.32		
PCO_2, mmHg	35–45	59		
HCO_3, mEq/L	21–28	28		
PO_2, mmHg	80–100	72		
O_2 sat, %	95–100	78		
Base excess, mEq/L	0 ± 2	-2.8		

Hospital Days 2-6: Craig remained intubated and sedated in the ICU. He received his BID dressing changes with antimicrobial ointment which lasted three hours each. He underwent two sessions of physical therapy (PT) each day in addition to one occupational therapy (OT) session during dressing changes. The nutrition consult with revised tube feeding goals was completed in the morning of day 2. Nursing reported Craig was advanced to your tube feeding goal later in the day on day 2 as had been tolerating the feeds well. His abdomen was reported to be soft and nondistended; however, Craig only had one bowel movement over a period of three days. Several liters of intravenous fluid (IVF) consisting of various solutions including lactated ringer's, D5NS with lytes, and 5% albumin were administered each day to keep Craig's urinary output at an average of 75 mL/hr. Medications during this time included wound healing micronutrient supplementation, morphine sulphate, fentanyl, lorazepam, a low dose of dopamine, SSI (receiving an average of 18 units per day); antibiotics including gentamicin, amikacin, and cefazolin; nebulized albuterol, heparin, and mucomyst.

Day 7: Craig was scheduled to go to the OR later in the day for wound debridement and allografting. Since Craig's respiratory status had started to improve, a metabolic cart study was completed at noon (prior to any daily PT or OT). Indirect calorimetry results indicate Craig had a resting energy expenditure (REE) of 2892 kcal/d and a respiratory quotient (RQ) of 0.86. Standard deviation of the REE is 147 kcal and of the RQ is 0.02. Measures indicate a steady state had been achieved. Craig's tube feeding was held at 3:00 p.m. and Craig was taken to the OR at 6:00 p.m. for the procedure that lasted four hours. He was admitted back to the ICU immediately post-op and the tube feeding resumed at goal rate once Craig returned to his room. Several liters of IVF consisting of various solutions including D5NS with lytes and 5% albumin were administered to keep Craig's urinary output at an average of 75 mL/hr. No bowel movement was noted. Additional IV fluids were provided during surgery. Medications on day 7 included wound healing micronutrient supplementation, morphine sulphate, fentanyl, lorazepam, a low dose of dopamine, SSI (receiving an average of 18 units per day); antibiotics including gentamicin, amikacin, and cefazolin; nebulized albuterol, heparin, and mucomyst. Daily Dulcolax was added to Craig's medications on day 7. Dressing changes using an antimicrobial ointment resumed BID post-op.

Hospital Days 8-30: Craig remained intubated and sedated in the ICU. He received his BID dressing changes with antimicrobial ointment which lasted three to four hours each. He underwent two sessions of PT each day in addition to one OT session during dressing changes. You continued to monitor Craig's tolerance to enteral nutrition support and provided appropriate follow-up progress and made additional suggestions based on Craig's status. Craig underwent surgical wound debridement and allografting on day 16. He received a tracheostomy at this time as well. A repeat metabolic cart study was performed on days 14 and 21. The results from day 14 were comparable to the results on day 7. The results on day 21 showed Craig had an REE of 2415 kcal/d and an RQ of 0.82. Standard deviation of the REE was 377 kcal and of the RQ was 0.27. Measures indicate a steady state had not been achieved. On days 20, 23, and 27, Craig had undergone more surgical debridement including allografting and autografting to the back and legs plus autografting to the hands. Craig was agitated most of the night after this last surgical procedure. He pulled out his nasoduodenal feeding tube twice during the night and therefore received a lower volume of enteral feeds. During this time, Craig's wounds were reported to show no signs of infection and contain some granulation tissue during inspection at dressing changes and surgical procedures.

Table 10.5: Comprehensive Metabolic Panel Obtained on Days 8 and 14.

Laboratory Value	Normal Ranges or Values	Craig's Laboratory Values Day 8	Craig's Laboratory Values Day 14	Craig's Trend (Improving, Stable, Worsening)	Implications or Assessment
Glucose, mg/dL	70–110	148	153		
Sodium, mEq/L	136–145	138	141		
Potassium, mEq/L	3.5–5.0	4.0	3.7		
Chloride, mEq/L	98–106	99	101		
CO_2, mEq/L	23–30	32	29		
BUN, mg/dL	10–20	18	16		
Creatinine, mg/dL	Male: 0.6–1.2	0.9	0.6		
Calcium, mg/dL	9.0–10.5	9.1	9.3		
Albumin, g/dL	3.5–5.0	3.0	3.1		
Total protein, g/dL	6.4–8.3	6.0	6.2		
Globulin, g/dL	2.3–3.4	3.6	2.9		
Bilirubin, total, mg/dL	0.3–1.0	0.7	1.0		
ALP, U/L	30–120	103	96		
ALT, U/L	4–36	32	30		
AST, U/L	0–35	31	28		

Table 10.6: Selected Values from Complete Blood Count and Differential Obtained on Days 8 and 14.

Laboratory Value	Normal Ranges or Values	Craig's Laboratory Values Day 8	Craig's Laboratory Values Day 14	Craig's Trend (Improving, Stable, Worsening)	Implications or Assessment
Hemoglobin, g/dL	Male: 14–18	12	14		
Hematocrit, %	Male: 42–52	43	45		
WBC, SI units	5–10	14.5	12.3		
Platelet count SI units	150–400	197	205		

Table 10.7: Selected Additional Labs Obtained on Days 8 and 14.

Laboratory Value	Normal Ranges or Values	Craig's Laboratory Values Day 8	Craig's Laboratory Values Day 14	Craig's Trend (Improving, Stable, Worsening)	Implications or Assessment
Prealbumin, mg/dL	15–36	7	9		
CRP, mg/dL	<1.0	55	77		
INR	0.8–1.1	1.0	1.1		
Phosphorus, mg/dL	3.0–4.5	3.5	3.3		
Magnesium, mEq/dL	1.3–2.1	1.4	1.9		

Overall during this time, nursing reported Craig tolerated your tube feeding goal well. His abdomen was reported to be soft and nondistended; however, Craig alternated between episodes of diarrhea and no bowel movements for days. Craig continued to receive several liters of IV fluids consisting of various solutions including lactated ringer's, D5NS with lytes, and 5% albumin to maintain adequate urine output. Medications during this time included wound healing micronutrient supplementation, morphine sulphate, fentanyl, lorazepam, a low dose of dopamine, SSI (receiving an average of 24 units per day); Dulcolax antibiotics including gentamicin, amikacin, and cefazolin; nebulized albuterol, heparin, and mucomyst. Dressing changes using an antimicrobial ointment continued BID. On day 10, oxandrolone was added to Craig's daily medications.

Hospital Days 31–45: Craig is continuing to improve. He continued to receive his BID dressing changes with antimicrobial ointment which lasted two hours each. He underwent two sessions of PT each day in addition to one OT session during dressing changes. He underwent several more surgical debridement and autografting procedures. The surgeons note Craig's wounds continue to improve, show no signs of infection, and are granulating well. Autografts have taken and most wounds are considered closed. Craig continued to tolerate his tube feeding well; issues with constipation and diarrhea are no longer present. Craig continued to receive several liters of IV fluids consisting of various solutions including lactated ringer's and D5NS with electrolytes to maintain adequate urine output.

On day 40, Craig was successfully weaned from the ventilator. Craig was happy to be off the "breathing machine" and wanted to eat. Craig successfully passed a swallow evaluation and was allowed to take an oral diet as tolerated. His overall intake of solid food was low; 10%–15% of each meal, therefore Craig remained on tube feedings. Craig complained of thirst and took po fluids well. Craig primarily wanted to drink water and became upset with his doctor and nurse when they started to limit water consumption; allowing for tomato juice, milkshakes or electrolyte replacement beverages.

During this time, the surgeon has been following your nutrition recommendations and Craig is doing well from a nutritional standpoint; tolerating nutritional intake from both oral intake and enteral support. His issues with constipation and diarrhea are no longer present. Medications during this time include wound healing micronutrient supplementation, morphine sulphate, fentanyl, lorazepam, Dulcolax, oxandrolone, ssi (receiving an average of 22 units per day); nebulized albuterol and mucomyst. Dressing changes using an antimicrobial ointment continued once daily. Craig was discharged to a rehabilitative facility on day 45.

Table 10.8: Comprehensive Metabolic Panel and Additional Labs Obtained on Days 28 and 41.

Laboratory Value	Normal Ranges or Values	Craig's Laboratory Values Day 28	Craig's Laboratory Values Day 42	Craig's Trend (Improving, Stable, Worsening)	Implications or Assessment
Glucose, mg/dL	70–110	165	151		
Sodium, mEq/L	136–145	143	139		
Potassium, mEq/L	3.5–5.0	4.4	4.7		
Chloride, mEq/L	98–106	100	99		
CO_2, mEq/L	23–30	29	26		
BUN, mg/dL	10–20	18	16		
Creatinine, mg/dL	Male: 0.6–1.2	0.8	0.8		
Calcium, mg/dL	9.0–10.5	9.8	9.5		
Albumin, g/dL	3.5–5.0	3.3	3.4		
Total protein, g/dL	6.4–8.3	6.2	6.5		
Globulin, g/dL	2.3–3.4	3.9	2.9		
Bilirubin, total, mg/dL	0.3–1.0	1.1	1.0		
ALP, U/L	30–120	96	88		
ALT, U/L	4–36	31	23		
AST, U/L	0–35	29	30		
Prealbumin, mg/dL	15–36	11	13		
CRP, mg/dL	<1.0–4.9	62	46		
Phosphorus, mg/dL	3.0–4.5	4.1	4.0		
Magnesium, mEq/dL	1.3–2.1	1.7	1.9		

Table 10.9: Selected Values from Complete Blood Count and Differential Obtained on Days 28 and 41.

Laboratory Value	Normal Ranges or Values	Craig's Laboratory Values Day 28	Craig's Laboratory Values Day 41	Craig's Trend (Improving, Stable, Worsening)	Implications or Assessment
Hemoglobin, g/dL	Male: 14–18	13	16		
Hematocrit, %	Male: 42–52	41	46		
WBC, SI units	5–10	10.5	9.3		
Platelet count SI units	150–400	198	285		

Table 10.10: ABG's Obtained after Weaning from the Ventilator on Day 40.

Lab Values	Normal Range	Craig's Laboratory Values	Craig's Value (WNL, High or Low)	Implications or Assessment
pH	7.35–7.45	7.39		
PCO$_2$ mmHg	35–45	44		
HCO$_3$, mEq/L	21–28	24		
PO$_2$, mmHg	80–100	92		
O$_2$ sat, %	95–100	97		
Base excess, mEq/L	0 ± 2	0.3		

Case Evaluation

Prioritize Problems and Identify Interprofessional Care

1. List in order of importance Craig's medical/nutritional concerns from admit date through hospital day 2.

2. Review the concerns listed in question 1. Which member of the healthcare team should address each concern and how should the concern be addressed?

3. List in order of importance Craig's medical/nutritional concerns on hospital day 7.

4. Review the concerns listed in question 3. Which member of the healthcare team should address each concern and how should the concern be addressed?

5. List in order of importance Craig's medical/nutritional concerns on hospital day 21.

6. Review the concerns listed in question 5. Which member of the healthcare team should address each concern and how should the concern be addressed?

7. List in order of importance Craig's medical/nutritional concerns on hospital day 43.

8. Review the concerns listed in question 7. Which member of the healthcare team should address each concern and how should the concern be addressed?

Disease/Injury Process and Laboratory Interpretation

9. Are there laboratory values or vital signs that would be a concern regarding Craig's condition upon admit to the hospital?

10. When reviewing Craig's ABG's upon admit to the hospital, what is your overall assessment of his acid–base balance?

11. Would adverse gastrointestinal (GI) symptoms be expected with a burn and inhalational injury? Would tolerance to enteral feeds be expected? Explain.

12. **a.** What is the Parkland formula and why is it used?

    b. Calculate Craig's twenty-four-hour resuscitation fluid needs based on the Parkland formula.

13. Craig was in the hospital for over six weeks. Several sets of labs were drawn. Describe some unique patterns/trends you see in his labs and your evaluation of why these occurred.

Anthropometric and Nutrition Assessment

14. What is your evaluation of Craig's height/weight status upon admit?

15. What assumptions can you make about Craig's preinjury nutritional status? Are there any labs or clinical data that can support this evaluation?

16. During his hospital stay, Craig's weight fluctuated as noted in the following table. What is the significance of these weight changes and probable causes?

Table 10.11: Weight Changes over Hospital Course.

Hospital Day	Craig's Weight in kg	Weight Change	Describe Significance of Each Weight Change and Probable Causes
Stated weight	65.0		
Admit—ER	66.3		
Day 3	70.7		
Day 10	70.9		
Day 15	67.3		
Day 25	64.2		
Day 35	62.5		

17. **a.** Craig was admitted with a 48% TBSA burn and underwent Parkland resuscitation. Describe the challenges of obtaining body composition data using BIA with Craig.

   b. Describe how you would assess or evaluate Craig's body composition once he was admitted to his hospital room and you were able to thoroughly review his medical record.

18. Upon admit, can Craig be diagnosed with malnutrition based on the ASPEN/AND guidelines? Explain.

19. Is there a reason to expect Craig to have micronutrient deficiencies upon admit? Explain.

20. Calculate Craig's total energy requirements on day 2. Justify your reasoning for method to determine needs.

21. Calculate Craig's protein requirements on day 2.

22. a. What are Craig's total energy requirements based on the results of the metabolic cart study on days 7 and 14?

   b. Would you make any changes to protein requirements based on your assessment in 22a? Explain.

23. a. What are Craig's total energy requirements based on the results of the metabolic cart study on day 21?

   b. Would you make any changes to protein requirements based on your assessment in 23a? Explain.

Medications

24. Craig received multiple antibiotics while in the hospital. Diarrhea is one of the side effects of antibiotics. How would you address this issue if the MD was concerned about a "tube feeding causing diarrhea"?

25. a. Describe the main functions of dopamine. Describe any possible adverse side effects or drug–nutrient interactions with this medication.

b. Craig received the dopamine at a low dose. What would need to be done with the tube feeding if the dose of dopamine had to be significantly increased and was now considered to be "very high"? Explain why.

26. Craig received morphine and fentanyl for pain control. Describe GI side effects of these medications and how you would address these side effects.

27. Craig received lorazepam. Describe GI side effects of this medication and how you would address these side effects.

28. a. On day 10, Craig started to receive oxandrolone. What is the purpose of this medication?

b. What needs to be done with regards to nutritional support or dietary intake while a patient is receiving oxandrolone?

c. Describe potential drug–nutrient interactions or side effects from oxandrolone administration.

d. What labs must be monitored when a patient is receiving oxandrolone and why?

Nutrition Intervention and Recommendations

29. Describe additional micronutrient supplementation for burn patients. Indicate nutrient and doses. Are these supplements indicated when Craig is receiving full enteral nutrition support? Explain.

30. What is your initial tube feeding recommendation for Craig on day 2? Provide nutrition therapy recommendations by citing enteral product, goal rate/hr, and daily volume to be infused; total kcal, grams protein, ml free water, %RDI, and grams fiber, (if indicated). Refer to your answer in questions 20 and 21 above.

31. What changes to Craig's nutrition support therapy would you make based on the results of the metabolic cart study on day 7. Provide nutrition therapy recommendations by citing enteral product, goal rate/hr and daily volume to be infused; total kcal, grams protein, ml free water, %RDI, and grams fiber, (if indicated). Refer to your answer in question 22 above.

32. What changes to Craig's nutrition support therapy would you make based on the results of the metabolic cart study on day 21. Provide nutrition therapy recommendations by citing enteral product, goal rate/hr, and daily volume to be infused; total kcal, grams protein, metal free water, %RDI, and grams fiber, (if indicated).

33. **a.** Craig started to take an oral diet and fluids on day 40. Assume you are doing a follow-up on day 41. Describe the appropriate diet for a burn patient.

    b. What changes to Craig's nutrition support therapy would you make based on the advancement of Craig's diet considering his eating patterns by days 40–41? Provide nutrition therapy recommendations by citing enteral product, goal rate/hr, and daily volume to be infused; total kcal, grams protein, ml free water, %RDI, and grams fiber, (if indicated).

34. Craig was discharged to a rehabilitative facility on day 45. What would be your final discharge feeding recommendations you would like to send to the rehab facility?

35. What specific criteria would you like to see met before you would recommend changing Craig to supplemental nocturnal tube feedings?

36. What specific criteria would you like to see met before you would recommend stopping Craig's supplemental tube feedings?

Monitoring and Evaluation; Patient Follow-Up

37. How often should Craig's tolerance and response to his enteral feedings be evaluated during his hospitalization? Explain specifically how you would evaluate tolerance to enteral feeds.

38. Are there specific laboratory values you would like to obtain as part of your nutrition monitoring? Cite labs and explain why.

39. Once his diet is advanced, how often should Craig's tolerance and response to oral intake be evaluated? Please cite your recommendations and what would you monitor?

Academy of Nutrition and Dietetics (AND) Medical Nutrition Therapy (MNT) Guidelines and Documentation for Dietitians

Nutrition Diagnosis Utilizing the PES statements:

Day 2, Initial Consult

Day 7

Day 21

Day 43 in preparation for discharge to rehab

Nutrition Intervention and Goals Utilizing AND Terminology:

Day 2, Initial Consult

Day 7

Day 21

Day 43 in preparation for discharge to rehab

Nutrition Monitoring and Evaluation Utilizing AND Terminology:

Day 2, Initial Consult

Day 7

Day 21

Day 43 in preparation for discharge to rehab

REFERENCE LIST

American Burn Association. http://ameriburn.org/.

Charney, Pamela. "The Nutrition Care Process." *Pocket Guide to Nutrition Assessment*, edited by Pamela Charney and Ainsley Malone, 3rd ed., Academy of Nutrition and Dietetics, 2016, pp. 1–14.

Collier, Bryan R., et al. "Trauma, Surgery and Burns." *ASPEN Adult Nutrition Support Core Curriculum*, edited by Charles M. Mueller, 2nd ed., American Society of Parenteral and Enteral Nutrition, 2012, pp. 392–411.

Ireton-Jones, Carol, and Mary Kristofak Russell. "Food and Nutrient Delivery: Nutrition Support." *Krause's Food and the Nutrition Care Process*, edited by Kathleen Mahn and Janice L. Raymond, 14th ed., Elsevier, 2017, pp. 209–26.

Irving, Chelsea Jayne. "Comparing Steady State to Time Interval and Non–Steady State Measurements of Resting Metabolic Rate." *Nutrition in Clinical Practice*, vol. 32, no. 1, Feb. 2017, pp. 77–83.

Jenson, Gordon L., et al. "Nutrition Screening and Assessment." *ASPEN Adult Nutrition Support Core Curriculum*, edited by Charles M. Mueller, 2nd ed., American Society of Parenteral and Enteral Nutrition, 2012, pp. 155–69.

Malone, Ainsley, and Cynthia Hamilton. "The Academy of Nutrition and Dietetics/The American Society for Parenteral and Enteral Nutrition Consensus Malnutrition Characteristics: Application in Practice." *Nutrition in Clinical Practice*, vol. 28, 2013, pp. 639–50.

Merck Manual Professional Version. http://www.merckmanuals.com/professional/nutritional-disorders/nutrition,-c-,-general-considerations/nutrient-drug-interactions.

Nahikian Nelms, Marcia. "Metabolic Stress and the Critically Ill." *Nutrition Therapy and Pathophysiology*, edited by Marcia Nahikian-Nelms, 3rd ed., Wadsworth, Cengage Learning, 2016.

Nelms, Marcia, and Diane Habash. "Nutrition Assessment: Foundation of the Nutrition Care Process." *Nutrition Therapy and Pathophysiology*, edited by Marcia Nahikian-Nelms, 3rd ed., Wadsworth, Cengage Learning, 2016.

Pagana, Kathleen Deska, and Timothy J. Pagana. *Mosby's Manual of Diagnostic and Laboratory Tests*. Mosby/Elsevier, 2014.

Peterson, Sarah J. "Nutrition Focused Physical Assessment." *Pocket Guide to Nutrition Assessment*, edited by Pamela Charney, and Ainsley Malone, 3rd ed., Academy of Nutrition and Dietetics, 2016, pp. 76–102.

Turner, Krista L. "Pulmonary Failure." *ASPEN Adult Nutrition Support Core Curriculum*, edited by Charles M. Mueller, 2nd ed., American Society of Parenteral and Enteral Nutrition, 2012, pp. 412–25.

Van Leeuwen, Anne, and Mickey Lynn Bladh. *Davis's Comprehensive Handbook of Laboratory & Diagnostic Tests with Nursing Implications*, 6th ed., F. A. Davis, 2015.

Walker, Patrick F., et al. "Diagnosis and Management of Inhalation Injury: An Updated Review." *Critical Care*, vol. 19, 28 Oct. 2015, pp. 351. doi:10.1186/s13054-015-1077-4.

Winkler, Marian F., and Ainsley M. Malone. "Medical Nutrition Therapy in Critical Care." *Krause's Food* . Raymond, 14th ed., Elsevier, 2017, pp. 775–89.

Case Study: Trauma; Motor Vehicle Accident with Multiple Fractures and Internal Injuries

Case-Specific Learning Objectives

✓ Determine how different stages of injury, treatment, and recovery can affect nutritional requirements and intake.

✓ Develop and calculate parenteral and enteral nutrition support therapy.

✓ Interpret results of indirect calorimetry measurements to determine caloric goals.

✓ Understand how medications can affect feeding tolerance.

✓ Prioritize medical, surgical, and nutritional problems.

✓ Evaluate nutritional requirements and determine appropriate nutritional therapy when multiple medical and surgical concerns are present.

✓ Identify and calculate differences between acute care and rehabilitative nutritional requirements.

Our Patient: Scott K. is a thirty-eight-year-old male who is employed as a pilot for an airfreight company. He is married and has one teenage daughter. His widowed mother-in-law, a retired accountant, lives in the small guest house behind their home. Due to Scott's occupation, he has thorough physical exams every year. He had just underwent his annual physical exam last month and was noted to be slightly overweight, but in excellent health. At his last physical exam, Scott weighed 202 pounds and he is 6 feet tall. Scott enjoys a couple of beers each weekend and will go to a variety of restaurants with his family two to three times each week.

Medical and Surgical History: Unremarkable. Scott suffered the typical childhood illnesses, had a broken right arm at age 14 and suffered a concussion when playing high school football. Scott is allergic to penicillin.

Home Medications: None reported.

History of Current Events: Scott was driving home from the airport one evening and a drunk driver in a full-sized pickup truck traveling at an estimated speed of 100 mph t-boned Scott's SUV on the driver's side. Both the driver and passenger of the other vehicle passed away at the scene. Paramedics reported that witnesses to the accident noted Scott had lost consciousness in the accident, however he was awake but confused prior to their arrival on the scene. Due to the extent of damage to Scott's vehicle, it took firefighters over 1½ hours to free Scott from the wreckage. At this time, Scott was awake, appeared disoriented but responsive to questions. He reported his pain as a 10 out of a possible 10. Scott complained of a headache, left side abdominal pain, and left arm pain. The EMT's noted Scott had a Glasgow Coma Scale (GCS) score of 11. He had an obvious deformity of his left upper extremity. After extraction from the wreckage Scott appeared to be in respiratory distress. The EMT's nasally intubated Scott, placed him in full c-spine precautions, started IV fluids, and transported him to the nearest level 1 trauma center.

Emergency Room and Admit (Days 1–2): Scott was intubated, awake and confused when he arrived at the ER. A chest x-ray revealed a left flail chest involving four ribs and a hemopneumothorax. A left chest tube was placed and 200 mL of serosanguinous fluid was immediately drained. During this time, Scott received resuscitation fluids in the form of D5NS, lactated ringer's, and 25% albumin. Once Scott was stabilized in the ER, he was taken to radiology for an abdominal, chest, pelvic, and head computed tomography (CT) scan as well as x-rays of his deformed left upper extremity. X-rays confirmed Scott had a fractured left humorous in two separate places. The scan of Scott's head revealed a concussion. The pelvic scan was unremarkable but the chest and abdominal scans revealed a splenic laceration, a lacerated and fractured left kidney, a lacerated pancreas, and a perforated small intestine. It was incidentally reported that the muscle density around the L3, psoas muscle appeared "well defined and above average."

Scott was taken from radiology to the OR where an exploratory laparotomy was performed. The injuries to the spleen and left kidney were significant, so a splenectomy and left nephrectomy was performed. The pancreatic laceration was repaired. GI contents had spilled into the abdominal cavity. The surgeon removed 4 cm of the duodenum and 8 cm of jejunum. Remaining ends of the small intestine appeared "dusky," so the surgeon opted not to perform a reanastamosis at this time; the small intestine was left in discontinuity. The surgeon packed Scott's abdomen and left it open with plans to return to the OR for a "second look" in twenty-four to forty-eight hours. Scott was transported to the trauma ICU in critical condition early on day 2. Scott remained on mechanical ventilation. Standard post-op orders included a nutrition consult. Scott continued to receive fluids in the form of D5NS, lactated ringer's, packed red blood cells, and 25% albumin. A Foley catheter was placed to monitor urine output. Nursing reported adequate hourly urine output and a tender and firm abdomen. Post-op medications include morphine sulphate, fentanyl, propofol at 10 mL/hr, lorazepam, a low dose of dopamine, SSI, antibiotics including ciprofloxacin and metronidazole; and nebulized albuterol and mucomyst.

Table 10.12: Nonfasting Comprehensive Metabolic Panel, Osmolality, and Albumin/ Globulin (A/G) Ratio Obtained in the ER.

Laboratory Value	Normal Ranges or Values	Scott's Nonfasting Laboratory Values in ER	Scott's Value (WNL, High or Low)	Implications or Assessment
Glucose, mg/dL	70–110	215		
Sodium, mEq/L	136–145	140		
Potassium, mEq/L	3.5–5.0	3.9		
Chloride, mEq/L	98–106	99		
CO_2, mEq/L	23–30	28		
BUN, mg/dL	10–20	17		
Creatinine, mg/dL	Male: 0.6–1.2	1.0		
Calcium, mg/dL	9.0–10.5	9.4		
Albumin, g/dL	3.5–5.0	2.9		
Total protein, g/dL	6.4–8.3	6.1		
Globulin, g/dL	2.3–3.4	3.1		
A/G ratio	>1.0	0.94		
Bilirubin, total, mg/dL	0.3–1.0	1.1		
ALP, U/L	30–120	130		
ALT, U/L	4–36	43		
AST, U/L	0–35	44		
Osmolality, mOsm/ kg H2O	285–295	294		

Table 10.13: Selected Values from Nonfasting Complete Blood Count and Differential Obtained in the ER.

Laboratory Value	Normal Ranges or Values	Scott's Nonfasting Laboratory Values in ER	Scott's Value (WNL, High or Low)	Implications or Assessment
Hemoglobin, g/dL	Male: 14–18	14		
Hematocrit, %	Male: 42–52	42		
WBC, SI units	5–10	14.3		
Neutrophils, %	55–70	95		
Platelet count SI units	150–400	315		

Table 10.14: Selected Nonfasting Additional Labs and Vital Signs Obtained in the ER.

Laboratory Value	Normal Ranges or Values	Scott's Nonfasting Laboratory Values in ER	Scott's Value (WNL, High or Low)	Implications or Assessment
Prealbumin, mg/dL	15–36	12		
CRP, mg/dL	<1.0	31		
HgbA1C, %	<6.0	6.0		
INR	0.8–1.1	0.9		
Lactic acid, mg/dL	Venous: 5–20	20		
INR	0.8–1.1	1.0		
Phosphorus, mg/dL	3.0–4.5	1.8		
Magnesium, mEq/dL	1.3–2.1	1.1		
Amylase, Somogyi units/dL	60–120	205		
Lipase, SU/L	0–110	167		
Triglycerides, mg/dL	Male: 40–60	55		
Temperature, °F	96.4–99.1	101.4		
Blood pressure, mmHg	Systolic <120 Diastolic <80	80/50		
Pulse, beats/minute	60–100	95		
Respirations, breaths/minute	14–20	12		
Pulse oximetry, %	≤95	80		

Table 10.15: ABG's Obtained in the ER.

Laboratory Value	Normal Ranges or Values	Scott's Nonfasting Laboratory Values in ER	Scott's Value (WNL, High or Low)	Implications or Assessment
pH	7.35–7.45	7.33		
PCO_2, mmHg	35–45	48		
HCO_3, mEq/L	21–28	26		
PO_2, mmHg	80–100	75		
O_2 sat, %	95–100	80		
Base excess, mEq/L	0 ± 2	−2.1		

Hospital Days 3–5:
Scott remained stable, npo and intubated in the trauma ICU. He had a nasogastric tube (NGT) with approximately 600 mL of gastric contents draining every twelve-hour shift. On day 3, a nutrition consult for parenteral feeding suggestions was completed; parenteral feeds were initiated later that day. On day 4, Scott was scheduled to return to the OR for an abdominal washout and "second look." The terminal end of the jejunum looked a little dusky so an additional 3 cm of the jejunum was removed. The surgeon packed Scott's abdomen and left it open with plans to return to the OR for another look in twenty-four to forty-eight hours. Scott continued to receive fluids in the form of parenteral nutrition, D5NS, lactated ringer's, packed red blood cells, and 5% albumin. Nursing reported adequate hourly urine output and a tender and firm abdomen. Post-op medications included morphine sulphate, fentanyl, lorazepam, a low dose of dopamine, SSI (22 units provided daily); antibiotics including ciprofloxacin and metronidazole; and nebulized albuterol and mucomyst. Propofol was discontinued on day 5.

Hospital Day 6–7:
On day 6, Scott was taken to the OR for an abdominal washout and evaluation. The surgeon noted pink and healthy terminal ends of the small intestine so reanastomosis was performed. The surgeon was pleased with the appearance of the abdominal contents; all tissue appeared viable and there were no signs of infection; therefore, the fascia was closed but the skin remained open. The open area measured approximately 4 cm x 5 cm. A wound vac was placed on this open area at the end of the surgical procedure. The surgeon placed a nasoduodenal feeding tube while Scott was still in the OR. During this trip to the OR the orthopedic surgeon performed an ORIF (open reduction internal fixation) of the humorous fractures. Scott was transported back to the trauma ICU on mechanical ventilation. Post-op, a nutrition consult for enteral feeds was ordered. The surgeon noted that trophic feeds would be started early on day 7 with tube feeding advancement to start within twenty-four hours.

During this time, Scott continued to receive fluids in the form of parenteral nutrition, D5NS with electrolytes, packed red blood cells, and 5% albumin. Nursing reported adequate hourly urine output and a soft but tender abdomen. Medications included morphine sulphate, lorazepam, fentanyl, a low dose of dopamine, SSI (26 units provided daily); antibiotics including ciprofloxacin and metronidazole; and nebulized albuterol and mucomyst. Trophic tube feedings were started at 9:00 a.m. on day 7.

Table 10.16: Comprehensive Metabolic Panel, BUN/Creatinine, and A/G Ratios Obtained on Days 3 and 7.

Laboratory Value	Normal Ranges or Values	Scott's Laboratory Values Day 3	Scott's Laboratory Values Day 7	Scott's Trend (Improving, Stable, Worsening)	Implications or Assessment
Glucose, mg/dL	70–110	148	133		
Sodium, mEq/L	136–145	140	136		
Potassium, mEq/L	3.5–5.0	4.3	4.7		
Chloride, mEq/L	98–106	103	100		
CO_2, mEq/L	23–30	23	25		
BUN, mg/dL	10–20	22	35		
Creatinine, mg/dL	Male: 0.6–1.2	0.6	1.1		
BUN/creatinine ratio	10–20	36.6	31.8		
Calcium, mg/dL	9.0–10.5	9.2	9.3		
Albumin, g/dL	3.5–5.0	3.4	3.2		
Total protein, g/dL	6.4–8.3	6.4	6.2		
Globulin, g/dL	2.3–3.4	3.6	2.5		
A/G ratio	>1.0	0.94	1.28		
Bilirubin, total, mg/dL	0.3–1.0	0.8	1.0		
ALP, U/L	30–120	115	120		
ALT, U/L	4–36	33	33		
AST, U/L	0–35	33	35		

Table 10.17: Selected Values from Complete Blood Count and Differential Obtained on Days 3 and 7.

Laboratory Value	Normal Ranges or Values	Scott's Laboratory Values Day 3	Scott's Laboratory Values Day 7	Scott's Trend (Improving, Stable, Worsening)	Implications or Assessment
Hemoglobin, g/dL	Male: 14–18	14	12		
Hematocrit, %	42–52%	43	40		
WBC, SI units	5–10	9.5	9.3		
Platelet count SI units	150–400	175	185		

Table 10.18: Selected Additional Labs Obtained on Days 3 and 7.

Laboratory Value	Normal Ranges or Values	Scott's Laboratory Values Day 3	Scott's Laboratory Values Day 7	Scott's Trend (Improving, Stable, Worsening)	Implications or Assessment
Prealbumin, mg/dL	15–36	9	8		
CRP, mg/dL	<1.0	34	55		
Phosphorus, mg/dL	3.0–4.5	2.9	3.4		
Magnesium, mEq/dL	1.3–2.1	1.4	2.0		
Amylase, Somogyi units/dL	60–120	210	187		
Lipase, units/L	0–110	98	58		
Triglycerides, mg/dL	Male: 40–60	70	54		

Hospital Days 8–18: Scott remained intubated and sedated in the ICU. His prior medication schedule continued and he received IV fluids to maintain adequate urine output. He received a wound vac dressing change every other day. The surgeon noted the wound edges looked good with no signs of necrosis or infection. Overall good wound granulation tissue was noted with each subsequent wound vac change. Scott underwent a session of PT each day and sat up in the chair twice each day. Scott was advanced to his goal tube feeding rate by day 9 and the parenteral nutrition was discontinued. Scott's tolerance to enteral nutrition support continued to be monitored and appropriate follow-up suggestions were made based on Scott's status. The interprofessional healthcare team was pleased to see how motivated Scott was to cooperate with his treatment. Scott could write notes to his family and staff and stated he wanted to get off the ventilator, the tube feeding, and go to a rehabilitative facility soon. By day 16, the surgeon had started to wean Scott from the ventilator. During this time, Scott did experience some additional pain with breathing due to the healing flail chest.

Scott continued to receive fluids from D5NS with electrolytes. Nursing reported adequate hourly urine output, tolerance of enteral feedings, and a soft abdomen. Medications included a low dose of dopamine, SSI (18 units provided daily); antibiotics including ciprofloxacin and metronidazole; and nebulized albuterol and mucomyst. Scott received a patient-controlled analgesia (PCA) pump with morphine sulphate to assist with pain control.

Table 10.19: Fasting Comprehensive Metabolic Panel and Additional Labs Obtained on Days 8, 11, and 13.

Laboratory Value	Normal Ranges or Values	Scott's Laboratory Values Day 8	Scott's Laboratory Values Day 11	Scott's Laboratory Values Day 13	Scott's Trend (Improving, Stable, Worsening)	Implications or Assessment
Glucose, mg/dL	70–110	185	171	162		
Sodium, mEq/L	136–145	143	151	144		
Potassium, mEq/L	3.5–5.0	5.0	5.9	4.9		
Chloride, mEq/L	98–106	102	105	100		
CO_2, mEq/L	23–30	29	32	27		
BUN, mg/dL	10–20	48	73	47		
Creatinine, mg/dL	Male: 0.6–1.2	1.6	2.2	1.3		
BUN/creatinine ratio	10–20	30	33.2	26.2		
Calcium, mg/dL	9.0–10.5	9.9	9.9	10.2		
Albumin, g/dL	3.5–5.0	3.0	3.1	3.0		
Total protein, g/dL	6.4–8.3	6.0	6.3	6.0		
Globulin, g/dL	2.3–3.4	3.8	4.0	3.5		
A/G ratio	>1.0	0.79	0.78	0.86		
Bilirubin, total, mg/dL	0.3–1.0	1.7	2.2	1.3		
ALP, U/L	30–120	130	133	124		
ALT, U/L	4–36	37	32	30		
AST, U/L	0–35	40	38	33		
Prealbumin, mg/dL	15–36	14	17	12		
CRP, mg/dL	<1.0	43	88	62		
Phosphorus, mg/dL	3.0–4.5	4.6	4.9	4.2		
Magnesium, mEq/dL	1.3–2.1	2.7	2.9	2.0		
Amylase, Somogyi units/dL	60–120	180	157	125		
Lipase, SU/L	0–110	109	89	76		
Triglycerides, mg/dL	Male: 40–60	55	54	47		

Hospital Days 17–25: Scott was extubated from the ventilator on day 18. At this time, he required supplemental oxygen and additional morphine sulphate due to the healing ribs. Scott continued to receive a wound vac dressing change every other day with notations of good granulation tissue and an overall diminishing wound size by the surgeon. Scott continued to receive daily sessions of PT and he started to ambulate around the ICU with assistance of his nurse or physical therapist. He continued to tolerate his goal tube feeding and was advanced to sips and chips followed by additional liquids on day 20. Scott was allowed to start taking soft solid food of his choice by day 22. Scott's tolerance to enteral nutrition support continued to be monitored and appropriate suggestions were made based on Scott's status.

During this time, Scott continued to receive fluids from D5NS with electrolytes and po intake. Nursing reported adequate hourly urine output, tolerance of enteral feedings, and a soft abdomen. Medications included SSI (14 units provided daily); nebulized albuterol and mucomyst, oral Percocet and morphine sulphate via PCA pump. Scott was discharged to a trauma rehabilitative facility on day 25. At discharge, Scott still had the wound vac in place and was receiving enteral nutrition support. Discharge notes indicate plans to wean Scott off the tube feeding and plans for skin graft over the abdominal wound.

Table 10.20: Fasting Comprehensive Metabolic Panel and Additional Labs Obtained on Day 20.

Laboratory Value	Normal Ranges or Values	Scott's Laboratory Values Day 20	Implications or Assessment
Glucose, mg/dL	70–110	145	
Sodium mEq/L	136–145	143	
Potassium, mEq/L	3.5–5.0	4.0	
Chloride, mEq/L	98–106	100	
CO_2, mEq/L	23–30	25	
BUN, mg/dL	10–20	21	
Creatinine, mg/dL	Male: 0.6–1.2	1.0	
BUN/ceatinine ratio	10–20	21	
Calcium, mg/dL	9.0–10.5	9.6	
Albumin, g/dL	3.5–5.0	3.1	
Total protein, g/dL	6.4–8.3	6.1	
Globulin, g/dl	2.3–3.4	3.1	
A/G ratio	>1.0	1.0	
Bilirubin, total, mg/dL	0.3–1.0	0.7	
ALP, U/L	30–120	122	
ALT, U/L	4–36	31	
AST, U/L	0–35	30	
Prealbumin, mg/dL	15–36	16	
CRP, mg/dL	<1.0	23	
Phosphorus, mg/dL	3.0–4.5	4.4	
Magnesium, mEq/dL	1.3–2.1	2.0	
Amylase, Somogyi units/dL	60–120	100	
Lipase, SU/L	0–110	98	
Triglycerides, mg/dL	Male: 40–60	50	

Case Evaluation

Prioritize Problems and Identify Interprofessional Care

1. List in order of importance Scott's medical/nutritional concerns from admit date through hospital day 3.

2. Review the concerns listed in question 1. Which member of the healthcare team should address each concern and how should the concern be addressed?

3. List in order of importance Scott's medical/nutritional concerns on hospital day 9.

4. Review the concerns listed in question 3 above. Which member of the healthcare team should address each concern and how should the concern be addressed?

5. List in order of importance Scott's medical/nutritional concerns on hospital day 18.

6. Review the concerns listed in question 5. Which member of the healthcare team should address each concern and how should the concern be addressed?

Disease/Injury Process and Laboratory Interpretation

7. Are there laboratory values or vital signs above that would be a concern regarding to Scott's condition upon admit to the hospital?

8. When reviewing Scott's ABG's upon admit to the hospital what is your overall assessment of his acid–base balance? What is the primary cause?

9. Are there laboratory values on day 11 that would be a concern regarding to Scott's condition that may promote a nutrition therapy reevaluation? Clarify labs and your concerns.

10. Why were parenteral feeds initially prescribed for Scott? Do you agree with this nutrition therapy?

11. Scott suffered a traumatic injury to his pancreas. Follow the progression of his lab trends. Are there any precautions you needed to take with regards to nutritional therapy?

12. Scott suffered a traumatic injury to his left kidney and underwent a left nephrectomy. Follow the progression of his lab trends. Are there any precautions you needed to take with regards to nutritional therapy? Describe.

Anthropometric and Nutrition Assessment

13. What is your evaluation of Scott's preadmit height/weight status?

14. What is your overall interpretation of Scott's preinjury body composition? Does this assessment point to any nutritional concerns? Explain.

15. Periodic body weights were not obtained while Scott was in the ICU. Compared to Scott's preinjury weight, would you expect his ICU weights to be higher, lower, or the same as his preinjury weight as time in the ICU progresses? Explain the overall trends you would expect to see at various stages of Scott's ICU stay; example post-op, on day 11, etc.

16. Assume you are the receiving clinician at the rehabilitation facility where Scott has been transferred. Compared to Scott's assessed preinjury body composition, what changes would you expect to see in his body composition upon arrival at rehab? Explain why.

17. Upon admit to the ICU, can Scott be diagnosed with malnutrition based on the ASPEN/AND guidelines? Explain.

18. Do you feel Scott will be able to be diagnosed with malnutrition based on the ASPEN/AND guidelines later in his hospital stay? Explain.

19. Do you feel Scott will be able to be diagnosed with malnutrition based on the ASPEN/AND guidelines when he is admitted to the rehabilitation facility? Explain.

20. Calculate Scott's total energy and protein requirements on day 3. Justify your reasoning for method to determine needs.

21. Do you feel Scott needs additional micronutrient supplementation? Explain

22. How would you reassess Scott's total energy and protein requirements based on his labs on day 8? Justify your reasoning.

23. How would you reassess Scott's total energy and protein requirements based on his labs on day 11? Justify your reasoning.

24. **a**. Assume Scott develops acute kidney injury (AKI) on day 11 with subsequent worsening of his renal labs and status on day 13. How would you reassess Scott's total energy and protein requirements with the start of every other day hemodialysis treatments? Justify your reasoning.

    b. Assume Scott develops AKI on day 11 with subsequent worsening of his renal labs and status on day 13. How would you reassess Scott's total energy and protein requirements with the start of continuous renal replacement therapy (CRRT)? Justify your reasoning.

25. How would you reassess Scott's total caloric and protein requirements once he was ready to be discharged to the rehabilitation facility? Justify your reasoning.

Medications

26. Describe the main function of Propofol. Describe possible adverse side effects or drug–nutrient interactions with this medication.

27. a. Describe the main function of a low dose of dopamine. Describe possible adverse side effects or drug–nutrient interactions with this medication.

b. Scott received low doses of dopamine during his ICU stay. Assume his dose of dopamine was considered to be very high. Describe how this would impact enteral nutrition support.

28. Describe the main functions of ciprofloxacin and metronidazole. Describe possible adverse side effects or drug–nutrient interactions with these medications.

29. Describe the main functions of morphine, lorazepam. Describe possible adverse side effects or drug–nutrient interactions with these medications.

Nutrition Intervention and Recommendations

30. a. What is your initial 2 in 1 parenteral feeding recommendation for Scott on day 3? Refer to energy and protein needs cited in question 20. Provide recommendations by citing total grams of protein and CHO/day; grams/kg protein; glucose infusion rate (GIR); total parenteral nutrition (TPN) goal rate/hr.

b. Cite intravenous fat emulsion (IVFE) total volume infused; grams fat/kg and IVFE infusion rate and duration.

c. Cite total kcal from TPN and IVFE; % protein kcal, % CHO kcal, and % fat kcal; total volume infused.

31. Do you agree with starting Scott on parenteral nutrition support on day 3? Justify your reasoning.

32. Scott suffered a traumatic injury to his small intestine. When making enteral nutrition support suggestions after reanastamosis are there precautions you needed to take with regards to nutritional therapy? Explain.

33. a. What is your trophic tube feeding recommendation for Scott on day 7? Refer to energy and protein needs cited in question 20. Provide recommendations by citing enteral product, goal rate/hr and daily volume to be infused; total kcal, grams protein, ml free water, %RDI, and grams fiber, (if indicated).

b. What will your suggestions for parenteral feeds be while Scott is receiving trophic enteral feeds noted in question 33a?

34. What is your recommendation for goal tube feedings? Refer to energy and protein needs cited in question 22. Provide recommendations by citing enteral product, goal rate/hr, and daily volume to be infused; total kcal, grams protein, ml free water, %RDI, and grams fiber, (if indicated)

35. What changes to Scott's nutrition support therapy would you make based on the changes in Scott's labs assuming the initiation of hemodialysis on day 11? Provide recommendations by citing goal rate/hr, energy,, protein, ml free water, % RDI and grams fiber (if indicated). Refer to energy and protein needs cited in question 24a.

36. What changes to Scott's nutrition support therapy would you make based on the changes in Scott's labs assuming the initiation of CRRT on day 11? Provide recommendations by citing goal rate/hr, energy, protein, ml free water, % RDI and grams fiber (if indicated). Refer to energy and protein needs cited in question 24b.

Monitoring and Evaluation; Patient Follow-Up

37. How often should Scott's tolerance and response to parenteral feedings be evaluated? Explain specifically how you would evaluate tolerance to parenteral feeds and what labs you would suggest monitoring.

38. How often should Scott's tolerance and response to enteral feedings be evaluated? Explain specifically how you would evaluate tolerance to enteral feeds and what labs you would suggest monitoring.

39. Assume Scott develops AKI. How often should Scott's tolerance and response (including lab changes) to nutrition support be evaluated? Explain specifically what you would evaluate if:
    a. Dialysis is not initiated.

    b. Hemodialysis is initiated.

    c. CRRT is initiated.

Academy of Nutrition and Dietetics (AND) Medical Nutrition Therapy (MNT) Guidelines and Documentation for Dietitians

Nutrition Diagnosis Utilizing the PES statements:

Day 3, Initial Consult

Day 7

Day 23 in preparation for discharge to rehab

Nutrition Intervention and Goals Utilizing AND Terminology:

Day 3, Initial Consult

Day 7

Day 23 in preparation for discharge to rehab

Nutrition Monitoring and Evaluation Utilizing AND Terminology:

Day 3, Initial Consult

Day 7

Day 23 in preparation for discharge to rehab

REFERENCE LIST

American Trauma Society. http://www.amtrauma.org/.

Charney, Pamela. "The Nutrition Care Process." *Pocket Guide to Nutrition Assessment*, edited by Pamela Charney, and Ainsley Malone, 3rd ed., Academy of Nutrition and Dietetics, 2016, pp. 1–14.

Collier, Bryan R., et al. "Trauma, Surgery and Burns." *ASPEN Adult Nutrition Support Core Curriculum*, edited by Charles M. Mueller, 2nd ed., American Society of Parenteral and Enteral Nutrition, 2012, pp. 392–411.

Ireton-Jones, Carol, and Mary Kristofak Russell. "Food and Nutrient Delivery: Nutrition Support." *Krause's Food and the Nutrition Care Process*, edited by Kathleen Mahn, and Janice L. Raymond, 14th ed., Elsevier, 2017, pp. 209–26.

Jenson, Gordon L., et al. "Nutrition Screening and Assessment." *ASPEN Adult Nutrition Support Core Curriculum*, edited by Charles M. Mueller, 2nd ed., American Society of Parenteral and Enteral Nutrition, 2012, pp. 155–69.

Jones, Kaeton I., et al. "Simple Psoas Cross-Sectional Area Measurement Is a Quick and Easy Method to Assess Sarcopenia and Predicts Major Surgical Complications." *Colorectal Disease*, vol. 17, no. 1, Jan. 2015, pp. 20–26.

Malone, Ainsley, and Cynthia Hamilton. "The Academy of Nutrition and Dietetics/The American Society for Parenteral and Enteral Nutrition Consensus Malnutrition Characteristics: Application in Practice." *Nutrition in Clinical Practice*, vol. 28, 2013, pp. 639–50.

Merck Manual Professional Version. http://www.merckmanuals.com/professional/nutritional-disorders/nutrition,-c-,-general-considerations/nutrient-drug-interactions.

---.http://www.merckmanuals.com/professional/injuries-poisoning/traumatic-brain-injury-%28tbi%29/traumatic-brain-injury.

Nahikian Nelms, Marcia. "Metabolic Stress and the Critically Ill." *Nutrition Therapy and Pathophysiology*, edited by Marcia Nahikian-Nelms, 3rd ed., Wadsworth, Cengage Learning, 2016.

Nelms, Marcia and Diane Habash. "Nutrition Assessment: Foundation of the Nutrition Care Process." *Nutrition Therapy and Pathophysiology*, edited by Marcia Nahikian-Nelms, 3rd ed., Wadsworth, Cengage Learning, 2016.

Pagana, Kathleen Deska, and Timothy J. Pagana. *Mosby's Manual of Diagnostic and Laboratory Tests*. Mosby/Elsevier, 2014.

Society of Critical Care Medicine. http://www.sccm.org/Pages/default.aspx.

Turner, Krista L. "Pulmonary Failure." ASPEN Adult Nutrition Support Core Curriculum, edited by Charles M. Mueller, 2nd ed., American Society of Parenteral and Enteral Nutrition, 2012, pp. 412–25.

van Leeuwen, Anne, and Mickey Lynn Bladh. *Davis's Comprehensive Handbook of Laboratory & Diagnostic Tests with Nursing Implications*, 6th ed., F.A. Davis, 2015.

Wojda, Thomas R., et al. "Ultrasound and Computed Tomography Imaging Technologies for Nutrition Assessment in Surgical and Critical Care Patient Populations." *Current Surgery Reports*, vol. 3, no. 8, 2015.

Case Study: Inpatient Suffering from a Traumatic Brain Injury Undergoing Treatment with a Pentobarbital Drip

Case-Specific Learning Objectives

✓ Interpret results of indirect calorimetry measurements.

✓ Understand how medications can affect nutritional requirements and feeding tolerance.

✓ Identify and calculate differences between acute care and rehabilitative nutritional requirements.

Our Patient: Paul T. is a twenty-four-year-old single male college student who worked part time as a bouncer at a local bar. He is 6 feet tall and his usual weight was 185 pounds. He rented a house two miles from his parents and has two younger brothers and one younger sister. All are active and healthy.

Medical and Surgical History: No prior surgical or medical history; healthy.

Home Medications: Paul takes no home medications or over-the-counter supplements other than a morning "protein shake" as per his roommate.

History of Current Trauma: Paul was riding his motorcycle to work in the late afternoon when a car cut in front of him. To avoid hitting this car, Paul had to lay down his motorcycle. Paul was not wearing a helmet. Emergency medical services were on the scene within 10 minutes of the accident. Paul was evaluated and the EMT's noted he appeared confused with a GCS of 12. IV fluids were started, and Paul was transported in full c-spine precautions to a local level 1 trauma center within 10 minutes of the EMT's arriving at the scene.

Emergency Room and Admit (Day 1) Events: Upon presentation to the ER, Paul was evaluated and his GCS was noted to be 10. A deformed RUE was noted. X-rays revealed Paul suffered a fractured right radius, ulna, and clavicle. The clavicle fracture is stable and nonoperative. Road rash of approximately 6% TBSA on right upper extremity and shoulder was noted. Paul was stabilized and transported to radiology for a CT scan of the head and spine. Injuries noted on CT scan include a traumatic brain injury (TBI), skull and facial fractures, and subdural and intracerebral hematomas. No spinal injuries were noted and it was incidentally reported that the muscle density around the L3, psoas muscle appeared "dense, well defined and above average." Once the CT scan was completed, Paul's GCS rapidly deteriorated to an 8. Paul was orally intubated (mechanical ventilation) and had an oral gastric tube in placed before being taken to the OR. In the OR, the neurosurgeon performed an exploratory craniotomy, evacuation of the subdural and intracerebral hematomas, as well as placement of an external ventricular drain (EVD). Post-op, Paul was admitted to the Surgical and Trauma ICU in critical but stable condition. Medications include cefazolin sodium, mannitol, and propofol at an average rate of 14 mL/hr.

Table 10.21: Nonfasting Comprehensive Metabolic Panel and A/G Ratio Obtained in the ER.

Laboratory Value	Normal Ranges or Values	Paul's Laboratory Values: ER	Paul's Value (WNL, High or Low)	Implications or Assessment
Glucose, mg/dL	70–110	173		
Sodium, mEq/L	136–145	142		
Potassium, mEq/L	3.5–5.0	4.7		
Chloride, mEq/L	98–106	101		
CO_2, mEq/L	23–30	34		
BUN, mg/dL	10–20	14		
Creatinine, mg/dL	Male: 0.6–1.2	0.8		
Calcium, mg/dL	9.0–10.5	9.2		
Albumin, g/dL	3.5–5.0	3.0		
Total protein, g/dL	6.4–8.3	5.9		
Globulin, g/dL	2.3–3.4	2.5		
A/G ratio	>1.0	1.2		
Bilirubin, total, mg/dL	0.3–1.0	1.0		
ALP, U/L	30–120	100		
ALT, U/L	4–36	35		
AST, U/L	0–35	33		

Table 10.22: Nonfasting Selected Values from Complete Blood Count and Differential Obtained in the ER.

Laboratory Values	Normal Ranges or Values	Paul's Laboratory Values: ER	Paul's Value (WNL, High or Low)	Implications or Assessment
Hemoglobin, g/dL	Male: 14–18	12		
Hematocrit, %	Male: 42–52	40		
WBC, SI units	5–10	14.2		
Neutrophils, %	55–70	95		
Platelet SI units	150–400	375		

Table 10.23: Nonfasting Selected Additional Laboratory Data and Vital Signs Obtained in the ER.

Laboratory Values	Normal Ranges or Values	Paul's Values	Paul's Value (WNL, High or Low)	Implications or Assessment
Prealbumin, mg/dL	15–36	15		
CRP, mg/dL	<1.0	24		
HgbA1C, %	<6.0	5.1		
Phosphorus, mg/dL	3.0–4.5	2.8		
Magnesium, mEq/dL	1.3–2.1	1.4		
Temperature, °F	96.4–99.1	100.4		
Blood pressure, mmHg	Systolic <130 Diastolic <85	145/90		
Pulse, beats/ minute	60–100	115		
Respirations, breaths/minute	14–20	24		
Pulse oximetry, %	≤95	92		

Hospital Day 3: After remaining in critical but stable condition on day 2, Paul was taken to the OR in the morning of day 3 to have his fractured upper extremity repaired. Paul received an open reduction and internal fixation (ORIF) of the radius and ulnar fracture from the orthopedic surgeon. The plastic surgeon repaired the facial fractures, performed a tracheostomy, removed the oral gastric tube, and placed a duodenal feeding tube. Upon return to the Surgical and Trauma ICU, Paul remained intubated and sedated. His neurological status was stable with intracranial pressures (ICP's) running between 12 and 17 mmHg. Post-op, the MD ordered a nutrition consult for enteral feeding goals. Day 3 medications included analgesics, SSI (8 units over the last twenty-four hours), propofol at 16 mL/hr, Mannitol, and cefazolin sodium. D5W is running at 50 mL/hr and urine output was noted to be adequate.

Hospital Day 4: Paul has been receiving and tolerating the enteral feeding recommended on day 3. The rate had been advancing every six hours to your eventual recommended goal. Nursing reported a soft abdomen; positive bowel sounds and bowel movements as well as adequate urine output. Paul continued to receive analgesics, propofol at 16 mL/hr, SSI (8 units over the last twenty-four hours), mannitol, and cefazolin sodium. D5W is running at 50 mL/hr and urine output was noted to be adequate. By midevening, Paul's neurological status became variable with frequent spikes in his ICPs; some as high as 19 mmHg and his GCS decreased to 8.

Hospital Day 5: Paul had been having elevated ICPs all night (18–28 mmHg), his GCS decreased to 6 and he was exhibiting motor posturing. Standard methods to control the ICP's were not achieving desired goals, so at 6:00 a.m., the neurosurgeon decided to put Paul on a pentobarbital drip. The pentobarbital rate was ordered to run at a rate to keep the patient still with a "couple of twitches" per hour. The nurse reported Paul had a soft and nondistended abdomen. Nursing reported Paul continued to tolerate enteral feedings immediately following the initiation of the pentobarbital drip. Propofol was discontinued once the pentobarbital was initiated.

A metabolic cart study was ordered and completed at 11:30 a.m. as the neurosurgeon expected Paul to remain on the pentobarbital drip for at least four to five days. Indirect calorimetry noted the patient had a REE of 1457 kcal/d and respiratory quotient (RQ) of 0.87. Standard deviation of the REE was 92 kcal and of the RQ was 0.02. Measures indicate a steady state had been achieved. Paul continued to receive analgesics, mannitol, pentobarbital, SSI (6 units provided) and cefazolin sodium. The IV of D5W was decreased to 15 mL/hr and urine output was noted to be adequate.

Table 10.24: Basic Metabolic Panel and Osmolality Obtained on Hospital Day 5.

Laboratory Values	Normal Ranges or Values	Paul's Values	Paul's Value (WNL, High or Low)	Implications or Assessment
Glucose, mg/dL	70–110	145		
BUN, mg/dL	10–20	17		
Creatinine, mg/dL	Male: 0.6–1.2	0.8		
Sodium, mEq/L	136–145	145		
Chloride, mEq/L	98–106	104		
Potassium, mEq/L	3.5–5.0	4.7		
CO_2, mmol/L	23–30	24		
Osmolality, mOsm/kg H_2O	285–295	298		

Table 10.25: Selected Additional Laboratory Data and Vital Signs Obtained on Hospital Day 5.

Laboratory Values	Normal Ranges or Values	Paul's Values	Paul's Value (WNL, High or Low)	Implications or Assessment
Prealbumin, mg/dL	15–36	8		
CRP, mg/dL	<1.0	45		
Albumin, g/dL	3.5–5.0	2.0		
Phosphorus, mg/dL	3.0–4.5	3.5		
Magnesium, mEq/dL	1.3–2.1	1.7		
WBC, SI units	5–10	11.4		
Temperature, °F	96.4–99.1	101.6		
Blood pressure, mmHg	Systolic <130 Diastolic <85	135/90		

Hospital Day 11: Paul's ICP's had been steadily decreasing over the last few days and were WNL (average 12 mmHg) for twenty-four hours. The neurosurgeon started to decrease the rate of the pentobarbital drip twenty-four hours ago. The neurosurgeon discontinued the pentobarbital drip at noon on day 11. Paul tolerated this medication change well. Once the pentobarbital was discontinued, Paul frequently moved and at times appeared agitated; he was rarely lying still despite the administration of sedatives making a repeat reliable metabolic cart study difficult to obtain. Day 11 medications included analgesics, Midazolam, SSI (5 units provided) and cefazolin sodium. Propofol was not provided at this time. He continued to tolerate his goal enteral feedings. Nursing reported a soft abdomen with positive bowel sounds and bowel movements every two to three days while Paul received the pentobarbital. Paul had a large bowel movement this at 1:00 p.m. D5W was running at 20 mL/hr and urine output was noted to be adequate.

Table 10.26: Basic Metabolic Panel and Osmolality Obtained on Hospital Day 11.

Laboratory Values	Normal Ranges or Values	Paul's Values	Paul's Value (WNL, High or Low)	Implications or Assessment
Glucose, mg/dL	70–110	151		
BUN, mg/dL	10–20	18		
Creatinine, mg/dL	Male: 0.6–1.2	0.7		
Sodium, mEq/L	136–145	140		
Chloride, mEq/L	98–106	102		
Potassium, mEq/L	3.5–5.0	4.6		
CO_2, mmol/L	23–30	28		
Osmolality, mOsm/kg H_2O	285–295	288		

Table 10.27: Selected Additional Laboratory Data Obtained on Hospital Day 11.

Laboratory Values	Normal Ranges or Values	Paul's Values	Paul's Value (WNL, High or Low)	Implications or Assessment
Prealbumin, mg/dL	15–36	10		
CRP, mg/dL	<1.0	40		
Albumin, g/dL	3.5–5.0	2.3		
Phosphorus, mg/dL	3.0–4.5	3.4		
Magnesium, mEq/dL	1.3–2.1	1.9		
WBC, SI units	5–10	9.6		

Hospital Day 26: Paul was weaned from the ventilator on day 20 and he had been breathing on his own without difficulties. Unfortunately, the damage to Paul's brain was severe. The neurosurgeon informed his family that Paul will have some permanent deficits. Paul will currently track with his eyes, move his extremities, and make unintelligible sounds. Paul is unable to feed himself and will spit out or pocket food if it is placed in his mouth. All fractures are healing and there are no concerns related to their status. The family consented to the placement of a percutaneous endoscopic gastrostomy (PEG) feeding tube in anticipation of discharge to a rehabilitative and extended care facility. IV fluids were noted to be running at a rate to maintain adequate urine output.

Table 10.28: Basic Metabolic Panel and Osmolality Obtained on Hospital Day 26.

Laboratory Values	Normal Ranges or Values	Paul's Values	Paul's Value (WNL, High or Low)	Implications or Assessment
Glucose, mg/dL	70–110	135		
BUN, mg/dL	10–20	20		
Creatinine, mg/dL	Male: 0.6–1.2	1.0		
Sodium, mEq/L	136–145	144		
Chloride, mEq/L	98–106	100		
Potassium, mEq/L	3.5–5.0	4.5		
CO_2, mmol/L	23–30	27		
Osmolality, mOsm/kg H_2O	285–295	290		

Table 10.29: Selected Additional Laboratory Data Obtained on Hospital Day 26.

Laboratory Values	Normal Ranges or Values	Paul's Values	Paul's Value (WNL, High or Low)	Implications or Assessment
Prealbumin, mg/dL	15–36	12		
CRP, mg/dL	<1.0	32		
Albumin, g/dL	3.5–5.0	2.5		
Phosphorus, mg/dL	3.0–4.5	3.5		
Magnesium, mEq/dL	1.3–2.1	2.0		
WBC, SI units	5–10 × 109 /L (SI units)	8.6		

Case Evaluation

Prioritize Problems and Identify Interprofessional Care

1. List in order of importance Paul's medical/nutritional concerns from admit date through hospital day 5.

2. Review the concerns listed in question 1. Which member of the healthcare team should address each concern and how should the concern be addressed?

3. List in order of importance Paul's medical/nutritional concerns on hospital day 11.

4. Review the concerns listed in question 3. Which member of the healthcare team should address each concern and how should the concern be addressed?

5. List in order of importance Paul's medical/nutritional concerns on hospital day 26.

6. Review the concerns listed in question 5. Which member of the healthcare team should address each concern and how should the concern be addressed?

Disease/Injury Process and Laboratory Interpretation

7. Are there laboratory values or vital signs that would be a concern regarding to Paul's condition upon admit to the hospital?

8. **a.** Describe the Glasgow Coma Scale.

   b. What is the significance of Paul's GCS in the ER?

   c. What is the significance of Paul's GCS after it dropped to 6?

9. What is the purpose of the EVD? How will this benefit Paul?

10. What is the significance of placing an oral gastric tube and providing oral intubation for Paul?

Anthropometric and Nutrition Assessment

11. What is your evaluation of Paul's admit height/weight status?

12. What is the significance of the CT scan body composition analysis of the psoas muscle at the L3 level?

13. Upon admit, can Paul be diagnosed with malnutrition based on the ASPEN/AND guidelines? Explain.

14. Is there a reason to expect Paul to have any micronutrient deficiencies upon admit? Explain.

15. No additional body weights were provided for Paul during his hospital stay. What changes in body weight/body composition would you expect to see by hospital day 26? What is the reason for these changes?

16. Are you concerned that the MD did not order enteral nutrition support for Paul earlier than day 3? Explain.

17. Calculate Paul's total energy and protein requirements on hospital day 3. Justify your reasoning for method to determine needs.

18. a. Reassess Paul's total caloric requirements on hospital day 5 based on the results of the metabolic cart study after the pentobarbital drip was started?

    b. Would you make changes to protein requirements calculated in question 17? Explain.

19. Reassess Paul's total caloric and protein requirements once the pentobarbital drip was discontinued on hospital day 11?

20. How would you reassess Paul's total caloric and protein requirements on hospital day 26 after placement of the PEG tube and in anticipation of long-term care/rehab placement?

Medications

21. Initially Paul received propofol at an average hourly rate. How will this affect the nutrition support he receives? Explain.

22. Describe the main function of mannitol. Describe any possible adverse side effects or drug–nutrient interactions with this medication.

23. **a.** What effect does pentobarbital have on energy expenditure?

b. Explain how can pentobarbital affect tolerance to enteral feedings?

c. What should be monitored to determine if Paul is tolerating his enteral feeds once the pentobarbital drip/coma has been initiated?

24. Describe the main function of cefazolin sodium. Describe possible side effects or drug-nutrient interactions with this medication.

25. Describe the main function of midazolam. Describe possible side effects or drug-nutrient interactions with this medication.

Nutrition Intervention and Recommendations

26. What is your initial tube feeding recommendation for Paul on day 3? Refer to kcal and protein needs cited in question 17. Do not forget to assess the effect of propofol administration on your recommended enteral feeding product and goal rate. Provide recommendations by citing enteral product, goal rate/hr, and daily volume to be infused; total kcal, grams protein, ml free water, %RDI, and grams fiber, (if indicated).

27. You reassessed Paul's nutritional requirements in question 18 based on the results of the metabolic cart study on day 5 and the initiation of the pentobarbital drip. Provide revised nutrition therapy recommendations by citing enteral product, goal rate/hr, and daily volume to be infused; total kcal, grams protein, ml free water, %RDI, and grams fiber, (if indicated).

28. You reassessed Paul's nutritional requirements in question 19 after the pentobarbital drip was discontinued. Provide revised nutrition therapy recommendations by citing enteral product, goal rate/hr, and daily volume to be infused; total kcal, grams protein, ml free water, %RDI, and grams fiber, (if indicated).

29. Eventually Paul will receive a PEG tube and be discharged to a rehabilitative and extended care facility on full enteral feeds. You reassessed Paul's nutritional requirements in question 20 in anticipation of his discharge. Provide nutrition therapy recommendations by citing enteral product, goal rate/hr, and daily volume to be infused; total kcal, grams protein, ml free water, %RDI, and grams fiber, (if indicated).

Monitoring and Evaluation; Patient Follow-Up

30. How often should Paul's tolerance and response to his enteral feedings be evaluated while he is receiving the pentobarbital drip? Explain how you would evaluate tolerance to enteral feeds and what labs you would suggest monitoring.

31. What would you recommend if Paul becomes intolerant to enteral feedings while he is receiving the pentobarbital drip? Explain your rationale for this decision.

32. How often should Paul's tolerance and response to his enteral feedings be evaluated on and after day 11? Explain how you would evaluate tolerance to enteral feeds and what labs you would suggest monitoring.

33. The risk for duodenal feeding tube displacement and aspiration is higher on and after day 11 when Paul was reported to appear agitated. Describe precautions you would recommend minimizing the risk of Paul's feeding tube becoming displaced and potentially experiencing aspiration.

34. How often should Paul's tolerance and response to enteral feedings be evaluated while he is in the rehabilitative facility? Please cite your recommendations and what labs you would suggest monitoring.

Academy of Nutrition and Dietetics (AND) Medical Nutrition Therapy (MNT) Guidelines and Documentation for Dietitians.

Nutrition Diagnosis Utilizing the PES Statements:

Day 3, Initial Consult

Day 5

Day 11

Day 26

Nutrition Intervention and Goals Utilizing AND Terminology

Day 3, Initial Consult

Day 5

Day 11

Day 26

Nutrition Monitoring and Evaluation Utilizing AND Terminology

Day 3, Initial Consult

Day 5

Day 11

Day 26

REFERENCE LIST

Brain Injury Association of America. http://www.biausa.org/.

Brain Trauma Foundation. http://www.braintrauma.org/.

Chapple, Lee-anne S., et al. "Nutrition Support Practices in Critically Ill Head-Injured Patients: A Global Perspective." *Critical Care*, vol. 20, 2016, p. 6.

Charney, Pamela. "The Nutrition Care Process." *Pocket Guide to Nutrition Assessment*, edited by Pamela Charney, and Ainsley Malone, 3rd ed., Academy of Nutrition and Dietetics, 2016, pp. 1–14.

Costello, Lee Anne S., et al. "Nutrition Therapy in the Optimization of Health Outcomes in Adult Patients with Moderate to Severe Traumatic Brain Injury: Findings from a Scoping Review." *International Journal of the Care of the Injured Factor*, vol. 45, 2014, pp. 1834–41.

Flower, Oliver, and Simon Hellings. "Sedation in Traumatic Brain Injury." *Emergency Medicine International*, vol. 2012, 2012, Article ID 637171, 11 p. doi:10.1155/2012/637171. (Received 8 Mar. 2012; Revised 16 May 2012; Accepted 22 June 2012).

Garvin, Rachel, et al. "Emergency Neurological Life Support: Traumatic Brain Injury." *Neurocritical Care*, vol. 23, Suppl. 2, 2015, p. 143. doi:10.1007/s12028-015-0176-z.

Irving, Chelsea Jayne. "Comparing Steady State to Time Interval and Non–Steady State Measurements of Resting Metabolic Rate." *Nutrition in Clinical Practice*, vol. 32, no. 1, Feb. 2017, pp. 77–83.

Jenson, Gordon L., et al. "Nutrition Screening and Assessment." *ASPEN Adult Nutrition Support Core Curriculum*, edited by Charles M. Mueller, 2nd ed., American Society of Parenteral and Enteral Nutrition, 2012, pp. 155–69.

Jones, Kaeton I., et al. "Simple Psoas Cross-Sectional Area Measurement Is a Quick and Easy Method to Assess Sarcopenia and Predicts Major Surgical Complications." *Colorectal Disease*, vol. 17, no. 1, Jan. 2015, pp. 20–26.

Kuroki, Lindsay M., et al. "Pre-Operative Assessment of Muscle Mass to Predict Surgical Complications and Prognosis in Patients with Endometrial Cancer." *Annals of Surgical Oncology*, vol. 22, no. 3, Mar. 2015, 972–79.

Malone, Ainsley, and Cynthia Hamilton. "The Academy of Nutrition and Dietetics/The American Society for Parenteral and Enteral Nutrition Consensus Malnutrition Characteristics: Application in Practice." *Nutrition in Clinical Practice*, vol. 28, 2013, pp. 639–50.

Merck Manual Professional Version. http://www.merckmanuals.com/professional/nutritional-disorders/nutrition,-c-,-general-considerations/nutrient-drug-interactions.

---.http://www.merckmanuals.com/professional/injuries-poisoning/traumatic-brain-injury-%28tbi%29/traumatic-brain-injury.

Nahikian Nelms, Marcia. "Metabolic Stress and the Critically Ill." *Nutrition Therapy and Pathophysiology*, edited by Marcia Nahikian-Nelms, 3rd ed., Wadsworth, Cengage Learning, 2016.

Nelms, Marcia, and Diane Habash. "Nutrition Assessment: Foundation of the Nutrition Care Process." *Nutrition Therapy and Pathophysiology*, edited by Marcia Nahikian-Nelms, 3rd ed., Wadsworth, Cengage Learning, 2016.

Pagana, Kathleen Deska, and Timothy J. Pagana. *Mosby's Manual of Diagnostic and Laboratory Tests*. Mosby/Elsevier, 2014.

Peterson, Sarah J. "Nutrition Focused Physical Assessment." *Pocket Guide to Nutrition Assessment*, edited by Pamela Charney, and Ainsley Malone, 3rd ed., Academy of Nutrition and Dietetics, 2016, pp. 76–102.

Ruf, Kathryn, et al. "Nutrition in Neurologic Impairment." *ASPEN Adult Nutrition Support Core Curriculum*, Charles M. Mueller, 2nd ed., American Society of Parenteral and Enteral Nutrition, 2012, pp. 363–76.

Teigen, Levi M., et al. "The Use of Technology for Estimating Body Composition: Strengths and Weaknesses of Common Modalities in a Clinical Setting." *Nutrition in Clinical Practice*, vol. 32, no. 1, Feb. 2017, pp. 20–29.

van Leeuwen, Anne, and Mickey Lynn Bladh. *Davis's Comprehensive Handbook of Laboratory & Diagnostic Tests with Nursing Implications*, 6th ed., F. A. Davis, 2015.

Wang, Xiang, et al. "Nutritional Support for Patients Sustaining Traumatic Brain Injury: A Systematic Review and Meta-Analysis of Prospective Studies." *PLOS ONE*, vol. 8, no. 3, 2013, p. e58838. doi:10.1371/journal.pone.005883.

Wojda, Thomas R., et al. "Ultrasound and Computed Tomography Imaging Technologies for Nutrition Assessment in Surgical and Critical Care Patient Populations." *Current Surgery Reports*, vol. 3, no. 8, 2015.

Zupec-Kania, Beth, and O'Flaherty T. "Medical Nutrition Therapy for Neurologic Disorders." *Krause's Food and the Nutrition Care Process*, edited by Kathleen Mahn and Janice L. Raymond, 14th ed., Elsevier, 2017.

APPENDIX A

Patient Assessment Worksheet

Primary diagnosis: Example: Stroke with left sided weakness

Pertinent secondary diagnosis: Example: History of hypertension

Pertinent Data	Comparison to Standard (Actual Data, High, Low, Etc.)	Historical Trend	Stable, Positive or Negative Trend	Malnourished or Risk of Malnutrition	Address Now or in Future	Desired Change	Recom- mendation for Desired Change	Interpro- fessional Referral and to Whom
Nutritional Intake and History								
Example: 55 g of protein/day intake based on typical dietary intake	RDA = 65 g protein/day intake	Recall from 1 month ago = 55 g protein/day intake	Stable and negative	Possible risk. Need to check additional data	Now	Increase in oral protein intake	Add 2 protein shakes/day as snacks. Patient unable to increase food consumption at mealtimes	RDN to address. Refer to PT so protein shake is offered after each afternoon PT session

Pertinent Data	Comparison to Standard (Actual Data, High, Low, Etc.)	Historical Trend	Stable, Positive or Negative Trend	Malnourished or Risk of Malnutrition	Address Now or in Future	Desired Change	Recommendation for Desired Change	Interprofessional Referral and to Whom
Anthropometrics								
Nutrition Focused Physical Assessment Data								

Pertinent Data	Comparison to Standard (Actual Data, High, Low, Etc.)	Historical Trend	Stable, Positive or Negative Trend	Malnourished or Risk of Malnutrition	Address Now or in Future	Desired Change	Recom-mendation for Desired Change	Interpro-fessional Referral and to Whom
Laboratory								
Medications								
Example: Percocet for pain; c/o constipation	New Rx for 14 days	Chronic constipation not noted	Negatively affecting po	Risk present if po further decreases	Now	Regular BM's	Increase po water and add psyllium as tolerated	Speak to MD and Pharm D regarding bowel care and alternative medications

Pertinent Data	Comparison to Standard (Actual Data, High, Low, Etc.)	Historical Trend	Stable, Positive or Negative Trend	Malnourished or Risk of Malnutrition	Address Now or in Future	Desired Change	Recom- mendation for Desired Change	Interpro- fessional Referral and to Whom
Education, Lifestyle and Personal Influences								

Pertinent Data	Comparison to Standard (Actual Data, High, Low, Etc.)	Historical Trend	Stable, Positive or Negative Trend	Malnourished or Risk of Malnutrition	Address Now or in Future	Desired Change	Recom-mendation for Desired Change	Interpro-fessional Referral and to Whom
Nutritional Intake and History								
Example: 55 g of protein/day intake based on typical dietary intake	RDA = 65 g protein/day intake	Recall from 1 month ago = 55 g protein/day intake	Stable and negative	Possible risk. Need to check additional data	Now	Increase in oral protein intake	Add 2 protein shakes/day as snacks. Patient unable to increase food consumption at mealtimes	RDN to address. Refer to PT so protein shake is offered after each afternoon PT session
Anthropometrics								

Pertinent Data	Comparison to Standard (Actual Data, High, Low, Etc.)	Historical Trend	Stable, Positive or Negative Trend	Malnourished or Risk of Malnutrition	Address Now or in Future	Desired Change	Recom-mendation for Desired Change	Interpro-fessional Referral and to Whom
Nutrition Focused Physical Assessment Data								

Pertinent Data	Comparison to Standard (Actual Data, High, Low, Etc.)	Historical Trend	Stable, Positive or Negative Trend	Malnourished or Risk of Malnutrition	Address Now or in Future	Desired Change	Recom-mendation for Desired Change	Interpro-fessional Referral and to Whom
Laboratory								
Medications								
Example: Percocet for pain	New Rx for 14 days	Chronic constipation not noted	Negatively affecting po	Risk present if po further decreases	Now	Regular BM's	Increase po water and add psyllium as tolerated	Speak to MD and Pharm D regarding bowel care and alternative medications

Pertinent Data	Comparison to Standard (Actual Data, High, Low, Etc.)	Historical Trend	Stable, Positive or Negative Trend	Malnourished or Risk of Malnutrition	Address Now or in Future	Desired Change	Recommendation for Desired Change	Interprofessional Referral and to Whom
Education, Lifestyle and Personal Influences								

APPENDIX **B**

Developing Therapeutic Diets

Templates can be used to practice developing sample therapeutic diets or meal plans for specific populations.

Modified Consistencies Based on the Regular Diet

Appropriate conditions where a modified consistency diet would be recommended:

_____

The progression of food consistencies can be displayed in the following table:

Food	Blenderized or Straw Consistency	Pureed Consistency	Ground or Mechanical Soft Consistency	Regular Consistency
Breakfast items				
Example: Cereal	Cream of wheat with extra milk	Cream of wheat	Cheerios with milk	Homemade granola with milk
Midmorning snack (if applicable)				
Lunch items				

Food	Blenderized or Straw Consistency	Pureed Consistency	Ground or Mechanical Soft Consistency	Regular Consistency
Lunch (*continued*)				
Afternoon snack (if applicable)				
Dinner items				
PM snack (if applicable)				

National Dysphagia Diets

Appropriate conditions where these diets would be recommended:

_____

If a low sodium, low saturated fat or carbohydrate counting modification is needed, specify how you would further modify these dysphagia diets:

Food	Dysphagia Pureed	Dysphagia Mechanically Altered	Dysphagia Advanced	Examples of Further Modifications if Needed
Breakfast items				
Example: Fruit	Applesauce	Banana	Cantaloupe	½ cup applesauce (CHO counting)
Midmorning snack (if applicable)				
Lunch items				

Food	Dysphagia Pureed	Dysphagia Mechanically Altered	Dysphagia Advanced	Examples of Further Modifications if Needed
Lunch (*continued*)				
Afternoon snack (if applicable)				
Dinner items				
PM snack (if applicable)				

High- and Low-Fiber Diets

Appropriate conditions where these diets would be recommended:

_____

If a low sodium, low saturated fat or carbohydrate counting modification is needed, specify how you would further modify these fiber modified diets:

Food	High-Fiber Option	Low-Fiber Option	Examples of Further Modifications if Needed
Breakfast items			
Example: Fruit	Strawberries	Applesauce	1 ¼ cup strawberries (CHO counting)
Midmorning snack (if applicable)			
Lunch items			

Food	High-Fiber Option	Low-Fiber Option	Examples of Further Modifications if Needed
Lunch (*continued*)			
Afternoon snack (if applicable)			
Dinner items			
PM snack (if applicable)			

Added Calorie and/or Added Protein Diets

Appropriate conditions where these diets would be recommended:

Food	Added kcal Option	Added Protein Option	Added kcal and Protein Option
Breakfast items			
Example: Oatmeal	Oatmeal with added honey or butter	Oatmeal with added nonfat dry milk powder	Oatmeal with added butter and nonfat dry milk powder
Midmorning snack (if applicable)			
Lunch items			

Food	Added kcal Option	Added Protein Option	Added kcal and Protein Option
Afternoon snack (if applicable)			
Dinner items			
PM snack (if applicable)			

Lactose Free or Lactose Controlled Diet

Appropriate conditions where these diets would be recommended:

Food	Low-Lactose Containing Option	Lactose Free Option
Breakfast items		
Example: Three cheese omelet made with milk	Swiss cheese omelet, no milk	Omelet with veggies and no milk
Midmorning snack (if applicable)		
Lunch items		

Food	Low-Lactose Containing Option	Lactose Free Option
Afternoon snack (if applicable)		
Dinner items		
PM snack (if applicable)		

Gluten Free Diet

Appropriate conditions where these diets would be recommended:

_____

If a low sodium, low saturated fat or carbohydrate counting modification is needed, specify how you would further modify the gluten free diet:

Food	Gluten Containing Option	Gluten Free Option	Examples of Further Modifications if Needed
Breakfast items			
Example: Starch	Shredded wheat	Rice Chex	¾ cup Rice Chex
Midmorning snack (if applicable)			
Lunch items			

Food	Gluten Containing Option	Gluten Free Option	Examples of Further Modifications if Needed
Afternoon snack (if applicable)			
Dinner items			
PM snack (if applicable)			

Low FODMAP Diet

Appropriate conditions where these diets would be recommended:

Food	Higher FODMAP Foods	Low FODMAP Diet Option
Breakfast items		
Example: Fruit	Cherries	Blueberries
Midmorning snack (if applicable)		
Lunch items		

Food	Higher FODMAP Foods	Low FODMAP Diet Option
Afternoon snack (if applicable)		
Dinner items		
PM snack (if applicable)		

Antidumping, Gastric Bypass, or Gastroparesis Diets

Appropriate conditions where these diets would be recommended:

Food	Antidumping Diet	Gastric Bypass	Gastroparesis
Breakfast items			
Example: Scrambled eggs	Scrambled eggs	1 TB scrambled eggs	Scrambled egg whites
Midmorning snack (if applicable)			
Lunch items			

Food	Antidumping Diet	Gastric Bypass	Gastroparesis
Afternoon snack (if applicable)			
Dinner items			
PM snack (if applicable)			

Low Sodium, Low Fat, and Low Saturated Fat Diets

Appropriate conditions where these diets would be recommended:

_____

If a carbohydrate counting modification is needed, specify how you would further modify these therapeutic diets:

Food	Low Sodium Option	Low Fat Option	Low Saturated Fat Option	Low Sodium and Low Saturated Fat Option
Breakfast items				
Example: Cheese omelet	Omelet with low sodium cheese	Egg white omelet with low fat cheese and veggies	Egg white omelet with veggies	Egg white omelet with veggies and no added salt
Midmorning snack (if applicable)				
Lunch items				

Food	Low Sodium Option	Low Fat Option	Low Saturated Fat Option	Low Sodium and Low Saturated Fat Option
Lunch (*continued*)				
Afternoon snack (if applicable)				
Dinner items				
PM snack (if applicable)				

Carbohydrate Counting

If a low sodium modification is needed, describe how you would further modify these carbohydrate controlled diets: _____

Appropriate conditions where these diets would be recommended:

_____

Breakfast Items	G CHO	CHO Servings	G Pro	G Fat	kcal
Example: ½ cup Applesauce	15	1	0	0	60
Midmorning snack (if applicable)					
Lunch items					

Breakfast Items	G CHO	CHO Servings	G Pro	G Fat	kcal
Lunch (*continued*)					
Afternoon snack (if applicable)					
Dinner items					
PM snack (if applicable)					
Grand totals					

Laboratory Values: Significance and Nutritional Implications

Templates can be used to record nutrition-related information and implications of specific laboratory values.

Laboratory Value	Normal Values	Primary Indication of Laboratory Value	Increased Levels May Indicate	Decreased Levels May Indicate	Nutritional Factors
Example: LDL					
Low-Density Lipoprotein	<130 mg/dL	These lipoproteins are high in cholesterol and can form deposits inside blood vessels by increasing the risk of arteriorsclerotic disease	Cardiovascular disease, genetic hyperlipoproteinemia, excessive alcohol consumption	Genetic hypolipoproteinemia, hyperthyroidism	A high saturated fat diet may contribute to high LDL cholesterol

Laboratory Value	Normal Values	Primary Indication of Laboratory Value	Increased Levels May Indicate	Decreased Levels May Indicate	Nutritional Factors

Laboratory Value	Normal Values	Primary Indication of Laboratory Value	Increased Levels May Indicate	Decreased Levels May Indicate	Nutritional Factors

Laboratory Value	Normal Values	Primary Indication of Laboratory Value	Increased Levels May Indicate	Decreased Levels May Indicate	Nutritional Factors

APPENDIX D

Medications: Nutritional Implications and Drug–Nutrient Interaction Worksheet

Templates can be used to record nutrition-related information and implications of specific laboratory values.

Medication	Primary Use of Medication	Primary Action of Medication	Gastrointestinal Effects	Nutritional Considerations
Example: Lasix				
Generic: furosemide	1. Helps the kidneys to eliminate excessive fluid buildup in the body. 2. Used in patients who are retaining excessive amounts of fluid.	1. Inhibits renal reabsorption of sodium and chloride. 2. Water, sodium, chloride, magnesium, potassium and calcium are excreted in the urine.	May cause nausea, vomiting, anorexia, constipation and/or diarrhea.	Can increase the risk of developing dehydration and low blood levels of electrolytes that are excreted in the urine. (hyponatremia, hypochloremia, hypomagnesemia, hypokalemia and hypocalcemia)

Medication	Primary Use of Medication	Primary Action of Medication	Gastrointestinal Effects	Nutritional Considerations

Medication	Primary Use of Medication	Primary Action of Medication	Gastrointestinal Effects	Nutritional Considerations

Medication	Primary Use of Medication	Primary Action of Medication	Gastrointestinal Effects	Nutritional Considerations

Medication	Primary Use of Medication	Primary Action of Medication	Gastrointestinal Effects	Nutritional Considerations